Our sincere congratulations!

Your years of dedicated study will soon culminate in graduation. As part of Schering's tradition of concern for the professional pharmacist, we are pleased to provide you with this copy of the Pharmacy Examination Review Book.

We hope that it will help you prepare for your State Board Examination, and are confident that you will soon join the professional ranks of those serving the public in the vital role of Registered Pharmacist.

Jack Robbins

Jack Robbins, Ph.D., R.Ph.
Health Services Planning Manager
Schering Laboratories

P.S.
For information on Schering products or services, call (201) 931-2908 or write
Professional Services Dept., Kenilworth, N.J. 07033.

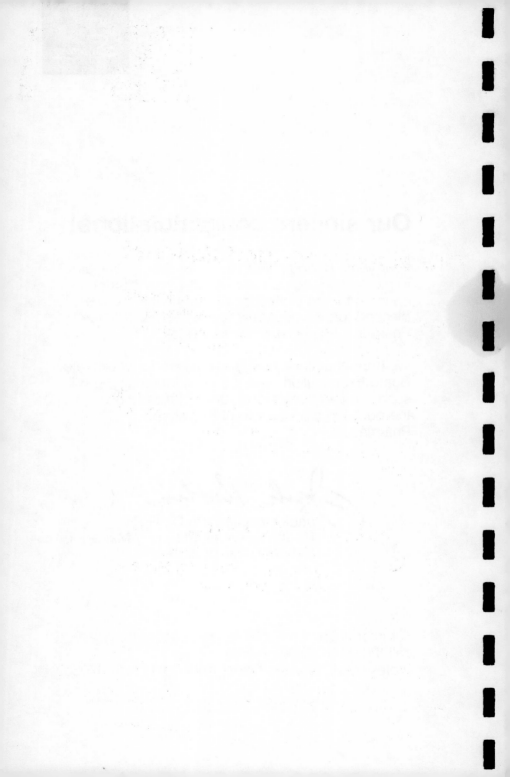

PHARMACY
EXAMINATION
REVIEW BOOK
VOLUME 1
SIXTH EDITION

2020 Multiple Choice
Questions and Answers

By

Robert J. Gerraughty, Ph.D.
Dean
School of Pharmacy
Creighton University
Omaha, Nebraska

MEDICAL EXAMINATION PUBLISHING COMPANY, INC.
65-36 Fresh Meadow Lane
Flushing, N.Y. 11365

PREFACE

There are no short cuts to the process of learning! The material on the following pages is not designed to provide the reader with an opportunity to escape from learning basic information that can only be obtained from textbooks. The purpose of this text is to encourage the reader to detect areas of weakness in his understanding of subject matter so that he may return to his texts for a more comprehensive review of the subject. Crossword puzzles are not designed to teach basic English; examination review books do not teach a basic understanding of the subject. However, the following pages will provide an interesting challenge to the student as well as an opportunity to improve his skills with multiple-choice examinations.

PHARMACY
EXAMINATION REVIEW BOOK

VOLUME 1
SIXTH EDITION

CONTENTS

FOR EACH OF THE FOLLOWING MULTIPLE CHOICE QUESTIONS,
CHOOSE THE ONE MOST APPROPRIATE ANSWER:

1. ACCORDING TO FDA, NITROGLYCERIN TABLETS SHOULD BE
   PACKAGED IN AMOUNTS NOT EXCEEDING:
   A. 100 tablets per container
   B. 50 tablets per container
   C. 500 tablets per container
   D. 200 tablets per container
   E. 25 tablets per container

2. EMULSIONS MADE WITH <u>TWEENS</u> ARE USUALLY:
   A. Unstable
   B. W/O
   C. O/W
   D. Clear
   E. Reversible

3. AMORPHOUS FORMS OF DRUGS ARE:
   A. Usually less soluble than crystal forms
   B. Usually more soluble than crystal forms
   C. Also called solvates
   D. Practically insoluble
   E. Usually less active than other metastable polymorphs

4. STREPTOMYCIN IS MOST SOLUBLE IN:
   A. Alcohol
   B. CHCl3
   C. Water
   D. Ether
   E. Pet. benzine

5. A ROLLER MILL IS USED MAINLY TO REDUCE PARTICLE SIZE IN:
   A. Tablet granulations
   B. Ointments
   C. Capsules
   D. Bulk powders
   E. Emulsions

6. PARTICLE SIZE REDUCTION WILL IMPEDE THE ABSORPTION OF:
   A. Hydrophobic compounds
   B. Hydrophilic compounds
   C. Weak acids
   D. Weak bases
   E. None of these

7. PARALDEHYDE IS A POLYMER OF:
   A. Formaldehyde
   B. Acetaldehyde
   C. Acetone
   D. Paraformaldehyde
   E. None of these

8. A LIQUID WHOSE VISCOSITY IS INCREASED WHEN STRESS IS APPLIED
   IS CLASSED AS A_____MATERIAL.
   A. Dilatant
   B. Newtonian
   C. Plastic
   D. Pseudoplastic
   E. Thixotropic

9. A SOLUTION CONTAINS 3 GR. OF A DRUG PER FLUID OUNCE. WHAT
   IS THE % W/V OF THE SOLUTION?
   A. 0.65%
   B. 0.59%
   C. 10%
   D. 1.0%
   E. 6.5%

10.   CYANOCOBALAMIN IS:
       A. A steroid
       B. A choline esterase inhibitor
       C. An hallucinogen
       D. A vitamin
       E. An enzyme

11.   IN STATISTICS THE MODE IS:
       A. The arithmetic average
       B. The midpoint of a series
       C. The same as the range
       D. The most common value found
       E. None of the above

12.   SPANS AND TWEENS ARE:
       A. Highly polymerized mannuronic acid anhydride
       B. Phospholipids
       C. Polyoxyalkalene derivatives
       D. Glycosides
       E. None of these

13.   WHICH OF THE FOLLOWING IS NOT A METHOD OF SPLITTING
       EMULSIONS?
       A. Centrifuging
       B. Filtering
       C. Addition of electrolytes
       D. Heat
       E. Addition of a liquid in which both phases are soluble

14.   IRON PREPARATIONS MAY STAIN THE URINE:
       A. Red   D. Purple
       B. Black   E. Brown
       C. Orange

15.   IF A YELLOW COLOR IS OBTAINED WITH SULFURIC ACID AND KI, THE
       IMPURITY PRESENT IS:
       A. Iodate   D. Iodide
       B. Potassium carbonate   E. None of these
       C. Nitrate

16.   WHEN PHENOL IS OXIDIZED, ITS COLOR IS:
       A. Black   D. Yellow
       B. Pink   E. White
       C. Brown

17.   IN PREPARING A PINT OF A 1:5000 SOLUTION OF $HgCl_2$, A PHAR-
       MACIST SHOULD USE_____MG.
       A. 190 mg.
       B. 95 mg.
       C. 19 mg.
       D. 9.5 mg.
       E. None of the above

18. ACETYLSALICYLIC ACID DISSOLVES WITH DECOMPOSITION IN:
    A. Alcoholic solutions
    B. Aqueous solutions of mineral acids
    C. Aqueous solutions of alkali hydroxides and carbonates
    D. Solutions of glycols
    E. None of these

19. RUTIN MUST BE PROTECTED FROM LIGHT BECAUSE IT CONTAINS A
    _____ GROUP WHICH BECOMES DISCOLORED.
    A. Phenol   D. Ester
    B. Hydroxy   E. None of these
    C. Catechol

20. THE TWO MAJOR PROPERTIES OF DRUGS THAT ARE USUALLY
    MODIFIED BY COMPLEXATION ARE:
    A. Odor and taste
    B. Taste and solubility
    C. Chemical structure and solubility
    D. Chemical structure and stability
    E. Stability and solubility

21. UNLIKE PENICILLIN, CHLOROMYCETIN IS:
    A. Water soluble
    B. Insoluble in alcohol
    C. Stable over wide pH range
    D. Insoluble in propylene glycol
    E. Unstable to sterilization

22. WHAT WILL RESULT IF THE DISTRIBUTION OF DRUG IS SLOWER THAN
    THE PROCESSES OF BIOTRANSFORMATION AND ELIMINATION ?
    A. High blood levels of drug
    B. Low blood levels of drug
    C. Synergism
    D. Potentiation
    E. Failure to attain diffusion equilibrium

23. THE TERM P. S. I. G. IN REFERENCE TO AEROSOLS MEANS:
    A. Propellant safety in glass   D. Atmospheric pressure
    B. Per square inch of glass   E. None of these
    C. Pounds per square inch gauge

24. IN RADIOPHARMACY THE TERM REM MEANS:
    A. Radiations per millisecond
    B. Radiations per minute
    C. Roentgen equivalent man
    D. External roentgens per minute
    E. Roentgen exposure per minute

25. TESTAPE IS USED TO DETECT:
    A. Pinworms
    B. Diphtheria reactions
    C. Sugar in urine
    D. Allergic reactions
    E. LSD

26. PHENOL IS:
    A. Soluble in water   D. Red in color
    B. Partially miscible in water   E. None of these
    C. A carboxylic acid

27. pH IS:
    A. Not temperature dependent   D. High for acids
    B. A measure of acidity   E. None of these
    C. The same as pOH

28. WHICH OF THE FOLLOWING TYPES OF TISSUES FREQUENTLY STORE DRUGS?
    A. Fatty tissue   D. A and B
    B. Muscle tissue   E. A and C
    C. Protein tissue

29. WHAT IS USUALLY THE FIRST EVIDENCE THAT A DRUG IS BEING STORED IN TISSUE ?
    A. Small apparent volume of distribution
    B. Large apparent volume of distribution
    C. Decrease of drug in urine
    D. Decrease of metabolites in urine
    E. Marked side effects

30. WATER FOR INJECTION DIFFERS FROM STERILE DISTILLED WATER AS IT:
    A. Contains sodium chloride
    B. Contains no pyrogens
    C. Is prepared by bacterial filtration
    D. May contain suitable preservatives
    E. None of these

31. WHICH OF THE FOLLOWING DRUGS UNDERGOES MARKED HYDROLYSIS IN THE GI TRACT?
    A. Aspirin
    B. Penicillin G
    C. Tylenol
    D. Hydrocortisone
    E. Chlortetracycline

32. SURFACE ACTIVE AGENTS TEND TO ENHANCE ABSORPTION DUE TO:
    A. Effects on biological membrane
    B. Effects on dissolution rate of drugs
    C. Reduction of interfacial tension
    D. B and C above
    E. A, B, and C above

33. _____ IMPARTS A PALE BLUE FLUORESCENCE TO URINE FOLLOWING ADMINISTRATION.
   A. Triamterene
   B. Cascara
   C. Riboflavin
   D. Azogantrisin
   E. Nitrofurantoin

34. WHAT EFFECT DOES PLASMA PROTEIN BINDING HAVE ON BIOTRANS-FORMATION?
   A. None
   B. Changes the mechanism
   C. Prevents formation of metabolites
   D. Slows the process
   E. Speeds up the process

35. A PATIENT SHOULD NOT EAT OR CONSUME ALCOHOLIC BEVERAGES FOR 24 HOURS PRIOR TO THE USE OF:
   A. Piperazine
   B. Hexylresorcinol
   C. Pyrvinium pamoate
   D. Indomethacin
   E. Tetracyclines

36. THE PRINCIPAL FACTOR THAT MAKES ENTERIC-COATED TABLETS UNPREDICTABLE IN DRUG THERAPY IS:
   A. pH
   B. Premature release of drug
   C. Failure to release drug
   D. State of health of patient
   E. Varying thickness of the coating

37. CARBOLIC ACID IS:
   A. Benzoic acid
   B. Aspirin
   C. Phenol
   D. Salicylic acid
   E. None of the above

MATCH THE FOLLOWING:

38. C Spansule   A. Schering
39. B Repetab   B. Abbott
40.   Enduret   C. S.K.F.
41.   Spacetab   D. Ciba
42. D Lontab   E. Sandoz

43. ANTITOXINS MUST CONFORM TO STANDARDS DISTRIBUTED BY THE:
   A. N.I.H.
   B. W.H.O.
   C. F.D.A.
   D. U.S.P.
   E. N.F.

44. TO OBTAIN A LICENSE FOR THE MANUFACTURE OF BIOLOGICAL
    PRODUCTS, THE MANUFACTURER MUST APPLY TO:
    A. The Surgeon General of U.S.P.H.S.
    B. U.S.P.
    C. N.F.
    D. F.D.A.
    E. N.I.H.

    MATCH THE FOLLOWING:

45. ___ Indomethacin   A. Povan
46. ___ Pyrvinium pamoate   B. Ilosone
47. ___ Erythromycin   C. Indocin
48. ___ Diphenhydramine   D. Lanoxin
49. ___ Ampicillin   E. Benadryl
50. ___ Digoxin   F. Polycillin
51. ___ Disulfiram   G. Antabuse

52. STERILITY TESTS FOR SUTURE MATERIAL REQUIRE INCUBATION FOR:
    A. 24 hours   D. 15 days
    B. 48 hours   E. None of these
    C. 7 days

53. STERILITY TESTS FOR MOLDS AND YEASTS SHOULD BE CONDUCTED
    WITH:
    A. Thioglycollate medium
    B. Agar plates
    C. Honey medium
    D. Glucose broth
    E. None of these

54. SOLUTIONS THAT CONTAIN BACTERIOSTATIC AGENTS:
    A. Cannot be tested for sterility
    B. Must be cultured on agar plates for sterility tests
    C. Must be diluted beyond the bacteriostatic level for sterility tests
    D. Do not require a sterility test
    E. None of these

55. THE STERILITY TEST FOR LIQUIDS INVOLVES:
    A. Colorimetric assay
    B. Rabbit test
    C. Injection into guinea pigs
    D. Culturing in fluid thioglycollate medium
    E. None of these

56. IN CARRYING OUT THE PRECIPITATION REACTION WHICH TAKES
    PLACE IN WHITE LOTION, THE SOLUTION OF SULFURATED POTASH IS
    ADDED TO THE ZINC SULFATE SLOWLY AND WITH CONSTANT AGITA-
    TION IN ORDER THAT:
    A. Polysulfides will not be precipitated
    B. Free sulfur will not be released
    C. A heavy precipitate will be formed
    D. A fine precipitate will be formed
    E. Basic salts will not be precipitated

57. STRONG IODINE SOLUTION CONTAINS KI FOR THE PURPOSE OF:
   A. Preservation
   B. Reducing agent
   C. Preventing precipitation
   D. Increasing potency
   E. None of these

58. DILUTED HYDROCHLORIC ACID HAS A STRENGTH OF:
   A. 20%
   B. 37%
   C. 1%
   D. 1 N
   E. None of these

59. LUGOL'S SOLUTION CONTAINS IN EACH 100 CC.:
   A. 9.5-10.5 gm. KI
   B. 25-250 gm. KI
   C. 15-25 gm. KI
   D. 5-15 gm. KI
   E. None of these

60. THE ADULT DOSE OF A DRUG IS 6 GR. WHAT DOSE, IN MG., SHOULD BE GIVEN TO A 6 YEAR-OLD CHILD ACCORDING TO YOUNG'S RULE?
   A. 195 mg.
   B. 10 mg.
   C. 65 mg.
   D. 100 mg.
   E. 130 mg.

61. WHY DOES THE U.S.P. STATE THAT MORPHINE SO_4 MUST BE KEPT IN TIGHT LIGHT-RESISTANT CONTAINERS?
   A. It loses water to the air
   B. It takes up water from the air
   C. It oxidizes slowly in air
   D. It takes up CO_2
   E. It volatilizes in air

62. A SOURCE OF ANTI-CARCINOGENIC DRUGS IS:
   A. Belladonna
   B. Nux vomica
   C. Vinca rosa
   D. Cascara
   E. Digitalis

63. AN Rx CALLS FOR 30 CC. OF A 1:500 SOLUTION OF ZINC SULFATE. WHICH OF THE FOLLOWING METHODS DOES NOT PROVIDE THE PROPER AMOUNT OF ZINC SULFATE REQUIRED?
   A. 2 ophthalmic tablets of zinc sulfate containing 1 grain per tablet
   B. 4.0 cc. of a stock solution 1:60 zinc sulfate
   C. 1 dram of a solution containing 8 gr./fl. oz.
   D. 2 tablets containing 0.030 gm. of zinc sulfate per tablet
   E. All provide the proper amount

64. IF A CNS DRUG IS EXTENSIVELY IONIZED AT THE pH OF BLOOD IT WILL:
   A. Penetrate the blood-brain barrier slowly
   B. Penetrate the blood-brain barrier rapidly
   C. Not penetrate the blood-brain barrier
   D. Be eliminated slowly
   E. Not be distributed to any tissue sites

65.   IN SITU SALT FORMATION IS A TECHNIQUE USED IN DRUG THERAPY
      TO OVERCOME:
      A.   Lack of solubility of salt
      B.   Complexation problems
      C.   Poor absorption
      D.   Chemical instability
      E.   None of the above

66.   ZINC SULFATE IS NOT INCOMPATIBLE WITH:
      A.   Soluble sulfides   D.   Lead acetate
      B.   Acacia   E.   Magnesium chloride
      C.   Pectin

67.   IF A DRUG HAS A BIOLOGICAL HALF-LIFE OF 6.9 DAYS, THE BEST
      DOSING INTERVAL WOULD BE:
      A.   Weekly   D.   Q.I.D.
      B.   Bi-weekly   E.   Daily
      C.   Semi-weekly

68.   TWEEN TWENTY IS A:
      A.   Deflocculant
      B.   Lipophilic surfactant
      C.   Preservative
      D.   Hydrophilic surfactant
      E.   None of these

69.   WHICH OF THE FOLLOWING FACTORS DOES NOT INFLUENCE THE RATE
      OF ADSORPTION FROM SOLUTIONS TO ANY SIGNIFICANT EXTENT?
      A.   Biological half-life   D.   Micellular solubilization
      B.   Viscosity   E.   Chemical stability
      C.   Reversible complexation

70.   FIRST ORDER HALF-LIFE IS EQUAL TO:
      A. $1/k$
      B. k D. $2k + 1$
      C. $0.693/k$ E.   None of these

71.   THE PURPOSE OF PARABENS IN SYRUPS IS AS:
      A.   Solubilizers   D.   Tonicity adjusters
      B.   Preservatives   E.   Thickeners
      C.   Buffers

72.   WHICH OF THE FOLLOWING IS NOT REGARDED AS A NARCOTIC?
      A.   Dionin
      B.   Meperidine
      C.   Morphine
      D.   Codeine
      E.   Propoxyphene

73.   BRIJ IS A TRADE NAME FOR A:
      A.   Suspending agent
      B.   Surfactant
      C.   Deflocculant
      D.   Propellant
      E.   Flavor

74. THE CONCENTRATION OF "DILUTED ALCOHOL" IS:
    A. 10%   D. 95%
    B. 50%   E. 20%
    C. 70%

75. A SUBSTANCE USED FREQUENTLY TO POLISH TABLETS IS:
    A. Sodium chloride   D. Starch
    B. Lactose   E. Calcium chloride
    C. Air dried talc

76. SODIUM LAURYL SULFATE IS:
    A. An alcohol   D. A wetting agent
    B. A ketone   E. A preservative
    C. A deflocculant

77. N.F. COD LIVER OIL:
    A. Must not contain any flavoring substance
    B. Must contain NLT 1% flavoring substance
    C. May contain NMT 1% flavoring agent
    D. Must contain added flavoring agent

78. A PRESCRIPTION CALLS FOR 25 MILLIMOLES OF POTASSIUM CHLO-
    RIDE. HOW MANY GM. OF KCl (M.W. 74.6) ARE NEEDED?
    A. 7.46 Gm.   D. 1.86 Gm.
    B. 0.746 Gm.   E. 0.186 Gm.
    C. 8.86 Gm.

79. AN I.V. ORDER REQUIRES 5 MILLION UNITS OF SODIUM PENICILLIN G
    TO BE ADDED TO A L. OF NORMAL SALINE. HOW MANY mEq OF
    SODIUM ARE AVAILABLE PER L. OF SOLUTION?
    A. 154   D. 162
    B. 1540   E. 1620
    C. 8.4

80. WHICH IS NOT CORRECT?
    A. Chloramphenicol is well absorbed by the oral route and diffuses well
       into tissues
    B. Solutions more alkaline than pH 9-9.5 are not stable and are rapidly
       destroyed
    C. Rectal doses of chloramphenicol for infants should be greater than oral
    D. Chloramphenicol is devoid of toxicity and is well tolerated
    E. An afebrile period follows administration of chloramphenicol in certain
       conditions

81. AN ORDER CALLS FOR 500 ML. OF A SOLUTION OF POTASSIUM SUL-
    FATE TO BE MADE SO THAT IT CONTAINS 10 mEq OF K+. HOW
    MANY GM OF POTASSIUM SULFATE ARE REQUIRED?
    A. 0.440   D. 0.870
    B. 4.44   E. 8.70
    C. 0.044

82. HOW MANY ML. OF A 10% KCL (M. W. 74. 6) SOLUTION CONTAIN 5. 0 mEq OF K^+ ?
    A. 2.10
    B. 21.0
    C. 3.73
    D. 37.3
    E. 0.373

83. GAMMA GLOBULIN FRACTION IS SEPARATED FROM SERUM BY:
    A. Centrifugation
    B. Filtration
    C. Dialysis
    D. Salting out
    E. Agglutination

84. THE OFFICIAL INSULIN UNIT IS BASED UPON:
    A. 1 hour frog method
    B. Blood sugar reduction in rabbits
    C. Blood pressure increase in dogs
    D. Lethal dose for cats
    E. Reduction of blood glycogen in dogs

85. HASHISH IS DIRECTLY RELATED TO:
    A. Opium
    B. Heroin
    C. Marihuana
    D. LSD
    E. Mescaline

86. TO ASSIST IN THE INCORPORATION OF PERU BALSAM INTO AN OINTMENT, THE FOLLOWING SHOULD BE USED:
    A. Alcohol
    B. Castor oil
    C. Solid petroxylin
    D. Glycerin
    E. Polyethylene glycol

87. TETRACYCLINES TEND TO FORM COMPLEXES WITH:
    A. Calcium ions
    B. Magnesium ions
    C. Aluminum ions
    D. Iron ions
    E. None of these

88. THE SPECIFIC GRAVITY OF ALCOHOL IS 0. 816 AT 15. 5° C., INDI-CATING 92.3% ALCOHOL. YOU DETERMINE THAT THE SPECIFIC GRAVITY BOTTLE HOLDS 48. 7 GM OF DISTILLED WATER. THE UNKNOWN ALCOHOL SOLUTION WEIGHS 39. 08 GM AT 15. 5° C. THE UNKNOWN ALCOHOL SOLUTION:
    A. Contains a higher concentration than is officially required
    B. Contains a lower concentration than is officially required
    C. Contains exactly 92.3% alcohol
    D. Has a specific gravity of 0.73
    E. Has a specific gravity of 1.227

89. _____ TEND TO INTERACT WITH ORAL DIURETICS.
    A. Pressor amines
    B. Dairy products
    C. Fish
    D. Chocolate
    E. Leafy vegetables

90. MOST DRUGS ARE:
    A. Strong electrolytes
    B. Weak electrolytes
    C. Non-electrolytes
    D. Highly ionic
    E. None of these

91. THE MAJOR MECHANISM OF DEGRADATION OF DRUGS IN THE GI TRACT IS:
     A. Oxidation
     B. Hydrolysis
     C. Acetylation
     D. Conjugation
     E. Reduction

92. THE MAXIMUM STORAGE TIME FOR INSULIN INJECTION AFTER
     LEAVING MANUFACTURER IS:
     A. 2 years   D. 6 months
     B. 5 years   E. Indefinite
     C. 2 months

93. AN ISOTONIC SOLUTION IS ONE WHICH:
     A. Does not cause hemolysis
     B. Has same salt composition of plasma
     C. Does not cause crenulation
     D. Causes crenulation
     E. Has a freezing point less than that of plasma

94. WHICH OF THE FOLLOWING DRUGS IS NOT DEFINED AS A NARCOTIC?
     A. Opium   D. Cannabis
     B. Dilaudid   E. Heroin
     C. Dihydromorphine HCl

95. WHICH OF THE FOLLOWING DOES NOT HAVE TO APPEAR ON AN Rx
     CALLING FOR TINCTURE OF OPIUM?
     A. Physician's signature
     B. Physician's telephone number
     C. Physician's address
     D. Physician's narcotic registry number
     E. Patient's address

96. THE BUFFER EQUATION IS ALSO KNOWN AS THE:
     A. Young's equation   D. Stokes' Law
     B. Charles' Law   E. None of these
     C. Henderson-Hasselbach equation

97. THE pKw OF WATER AT 25^{0} C. IS:
     A. 7
     B. 14
     C. 1×10^{-14}
     D. 1×10^{-7}
     E. 1

98. WHEN EXPOSED TO AIR, CITRIC ACID IS:
     A. Deliquescent   D. Partially volatilized
     B. Stable   E. Efflorescent
     C. Hygroscopic

99. ESTER HYDROLYSIS IS OF BENEFIT THERAPEUTICALLY WITH:
    A. Penicillin G
    B. Esters of erythromycin
    C. Esters of chloramphenicol
    D. A, B and C above
    E. None of the above

100. FOR WHICH OF THE FOLLOWING DRUGS IS BIOTRANSFORMATION ES-
SENTIAL FOR THERAPEUTIC ACTIVITY?
    A. Methanol   D. Aspirin
    B. Ethyl alcohol   E. Penicillin G
    C. Phenacetin

101. U. S. P. ACETYLSALICYLIC ACID TABLETS SHOULD BE PACKAGED AND
STORED IN:
    A. Well-closed containers
    B. Tightly closed containers
    C. Light-resistant containers
    D. Tightly closed, light-resistant containers
    E. None of these

102. CARON OIL IS:
    A. Lime liniment   D. Soap liniment
    B. Castor oil   E. Not a medicinal
    C. Olive oil

103. BENZALKONIUM CHLORIDE SOLUTION IS PARTIALLY
INACTIVATED BY:
    A. Soap   D. Acetone
    B. Warming the solution   E. None of these
    C. Methyl cellulose

104. THE USUAL PURPOSE OF CHILLING MEDICATION PRIOR TO ADMINIS-
TRATION IS TO INCREASE:
    A. Absorption   D. Ionization
    B. Palatability   E. Gastric motility
    C. Stability

105. A ROUTE OR METHOD OF ADMINISTRATION FOR DRUGS WHICH DIS-
TRIBUTE POORLY IS:
    A. I. M.   D. S. C.
    B. I. V. infusion   E. Intra-cerebral
    C. Tissue implant

106. A CHROMOGEN IS:
    A. Associated with heredity   D. A dye fixative
    B. A certified dye   E. A colored substance
    C. A precursor of color

107. HOW MANY GRAMS OF ASPIRIN MUST BE DISSOLVED IN 484 CC
OF ALCOHOL TO MAKE A 12% SOLUTION?
    A. 76   D. 48
    B. 66   E. 58
    C. 112

MATCH THE FOLLOWING INCOMPATIBILITIES:

108. _b_ Tannic acid   A. Hypophosphites
109. _C_ Elixir B1   B. Lime water
110. _A_ Mercurous chloride   C. Sodium phenobarbital
111. _E_ Mercurochrome   D. Copper salts
112. _D_ Epinephrine   E. Hydrogen peroxide

113. NEEDLE-SHAPED CRYSTALS ARE FREQUENTLY FORMED ON THE
     SURFACE OF ASPIRIN ON LONG STANDING DUE TO DECOMPOSITION.
     THE SUBSTANCE FORMED IS:
     A. $C_6H_4(OH)COOH$
     B. CH_3COOH
     C. $C_6H_4(OCH_3)COOH$
     D. C_6H_5OH
     E. $C_6H_4(OH)_2$

114. KEESOM FORCES OCCUR BETWEEN:
     A. Dipoles
     B. Induced dipoles
     C. Ions
     D. Ions and dipoles
     E. Ions and induced dipoles

115. EPHEDRINE IS SOLUBLE IN:
     A. Water   D. All of these
     B. Oils   E. A and B
     C. Alcohol

116. A ROBENGATOPE IS A RADIOISOTOPE USED PRIMARILY TO TEST:
     A. Brain function
     B. Kidney function
     C. Liver function
     D. Rate of excretion
     E. Rate of drug absorption

117. A SOLVENT WHICH CAN EITHER ACCEPT OR DONATE PROTONS IS
     SAID TO BE:
     A. Aprotic   D. Acidic
     B. Amphiprotic   E. Basic
     C. Proteolytic

118. GLYCERIN SUPPOSITORIES CONTAIN 92% GLYCERIN AND ARE SOLI-
     DIFIED BY THE USE OF:
     A. White wax   D. PEG 4000
     B. Stearic acid   E. Glyceryl triacetate
     C. Sodium stearate

119. WHEN SILVER NITRATE DECOMPOSES BY OXIDATION IT GIVES:
     A. A red precipitate   D. A green color
     B. A white precipitate   E. No visible change
     C. A darkened solution

120. THE K TERM IN THE BIOLOGICAL HALF-LIFE EQUATIONS IS A COM-
     BINATION OF:
     A. Ke and Km   D. Ka, Km and Ke
     B. Ka and Km   E. Ka - (Ke + Km)
     C. Ka and Ke

121. WHICH OF THE FOLLOWING IS NOT A MAJOR PATHWAY OR TYPE OF
     BIOTRANSFORMATION ?
     A. Oxidation   D. Hydrolysis
     B. Deamination   E. Conjugation
     C. Reduction

122. IN DISPENSING AZOGANTRISIN THE PHARMACIST SHOULD WARN THE
     PATIENT THAT:
     A. He is likely to get a rash
     B. The drug can only be taken at night
     C. The drug can only be taken in the morning
     D. It colors the urine red
     E. The drug should be taken with food

123. THE STRUCTURAL PART OF THE MORPHINE MOLECULE FOUND IN
     DEMEROL IS:
     A. Phenanthrene
     B. Piperidine
     C. Pyrimidine
     D. Pyrrole
     E. Pyridine

124. CLATHRATES ARE:
     A. Cage-like complexes   D. Pi bond complexes
     B. Chelates   E. Ligands
     C. Sandwich-type complexes

125. WHAT IS THE MAJOR REASON THAT ANIMAL STUDIES ARE NOT IN-
     FALLIBLE IN PREDICTING DRUG EFFICACY OR TOXICITY?
     A. Differences in biotransformation
     B. Differences in elimination mechanism
     C. Differences in distribution mechanisms
     D. Differences in absorption mechanisms
     E. Differences in average weights

126. TALCUM POWDERS ARE MOST EFFECTIVELY STERILIZED BY:
     A. Autoclave   D. Millipore
     B. Dry heat   E. Freeze drying
     C. Gas sterilization

127. THE U. S. P. PYROGEN TEST IS PERFORMED ON:
     A. Dogs   D. White mice
     B. Guinea pigs   E. Rats
     C. Rabbits

128. PLASTICS ARE NORMALLY STERILIZED WITH:
     A. Direct flame   D. Steam under pressure
     B. Oven heat   E. Steam under vacuum
     C. Ethylene oxide

129. SHRINKAGE OF GELS BY EXTRUSION OF LIQUID IS CALLED:
    A. Syneresis
    B. Coacervation
    C. Ebullition
    D. Dilatancy
    E. Plasticity

130. COMPAZINE SYRUP:
    A. Is deliquescent
    B. Is effervescent
    C. Should be dispensed in its original container
    D. Is hygroscopic
    E. Should never be given to children

131. HOW MANY ML. OF CONC. HCl (37% w/w) WITH A SP. G. OF 1.35
    SHOULD BE USED TO MAKE 4 FLUIDOUNCES OF A 5% (w/v) SOLUTION?
    A. .12 ml.
    B. 120 ml.
    C. 1.2 ml.
    D. 9 ml.
    E. 12 ml.

132. THE DOSE OF A DRUG IS 0.5 MG. PER KG. WHAT DOSE, IN GM.,
    SHOULD BE GIVEN TO A CHILD OF SIX WHO WEIGHS 44 LBS?
    A. 0.003 Gm.
    B. 0.033 Gm.
    C. 0.010 Gm.
    D. 0.100 Gm.
    E. 0.05 Gm.

MATCH THE FOLLOWING WITH THEIR ASSOCIATED INCOMPATIBILI-
TIES:

133. ___ Aminopyrine
134. ___ Icthammol
135. ___ Iodoform
136. ___ Nitrites
137. ___ Resorcinol

A. Forms wet mass when triturated with aspirin
B. Decomposed by exposure to air in direct sunlight
C. Solutions are pptd. by acid
D. Oxidizing agents produce red to violet color
E. Liberates iodine from iodides

138. OLEIC ACID IS:
    A. A saturated fatty acid
    B. An unsaturated ketone
    C. Photosensitive
    D. Official as a salt
    E. An unsaturated fatty acid

139. RANCIDITY OF A FAT IS DUE TO:
    A. Oxidation
    B. Reduction
    C. Neutralization
    D. Hydrolysis
    E. Saponification

SECTION I - PHARMACY

140. THE MINIMAL EFFECTIVE FLOW RATE OF AIR IN LAMINAR FLOW HOODS SHOULD BE NOT LESS THAN _____ CUBIC FEET PER MINUTE (c.f.m.):
   A. 10   D. 500
   B. 50   E. 1000
   C. 100

141. WHICH OF THE FOLLOWING COMPOUNDS OF UNDECYLENIC ACID IS MOST COMMONLY USED IN THERAPY?
   A. Zinc   D. Silver
   B. Magnesium   E. Mercury
   C. Manganese

142. A VITAMIN WHICH STAINS THE URINE IS:
   A. Vitamin D   D. Riboflavin
   B. Thiamine   E. Niacin
   C. Inositol

143. WHAT EFFECT DOES INCREASED TISSUE STORAGE HAVE ON BIO-LOGICAL HALF-LIFE OF DRUGS?
   A. Makes it erractic   D. Increases it
   B. Renders it meaningless   E. None
   C. Decreases it

144. A 30 VOLUME PEROXIDE CORRESPONDS TO:
   A. 3% by weight   D. 9% by weight
   B. 30% by weight   E. 99% by weight
   C. 30% by volume

145. THE MUNSELL SYSTEM IS ASSOCIATED WITH:
   A. Flavor   D. Color
   B. Odor   E. Incompatibilities
   C. Chemical classification

146. THE DOSE OF A DRUG IS 5 MG/KG OF BODY WEIGHT. WHAT DOSE SHOULD BE GIVEN TO A 110 LB. WOMAN?
   A. 2 grains   D. 5 grains
   B. 4 grains   E. 0.5 grains
   C. 500 mg

147. THE TWO MOST COMMON PROTEINS INVOLVED IN PLASMA PROTEIN BINDING ARE:
   A. Plasmin and albumin   D. Fibrin and plasmin
   B. Globulin and plasmin   E. Plasminogen and fibrin
   C. Albumin and globulin

148. KANAMYCIN SHOULD NOT BE USED IN COMBINATION WITH _____.
   A. Barbiturates   D. Tranquilizers
   B. Analgesics   E. Diuretics
   C. Antacids

149. DIURETICS TEND TO ENHANCE LITHIUM SALT TOXICITY DUE TO:
   A. Sodium depletion
   B. Potassium depletion
   C. Direct drug interaction
   D. Increased absorption
   E. Increased solubility of the lithium salts

150.   AN ORAL ANTIFUNGAL AGENT IS:
        A. Zinc undecylenate   D. Griseofulvin
        B. Tetrex   E. Sopronol
        C. Desenex

151.   A DISADVANTAGE OF SODIUM SACCHARIN AS A SWEETENING AGENT
        IS:
        A. Its bitter aftertaste
        B. Its solubility in water
        C. Its poor strength compared to glucose
        D. Its poor strength compared to dulcin
        E. Its toxicity

152.   RESPONSIBILITY FOR CONTROL OF DRUGS COVERED BY THE DRUG
        ABUSE AMENDMENTS FALLS UPON:
        A. DEA
        B. FTC
        C. FDA
        D. ICC
        E. None of the above

153.   NITROFURANTOIN (FURADANTIN) IS MOST ACTIVE WHEN THE pH OF
        THE URINARY TRACT IS:
        A. Neutral   D. 5.5 or less
        B. Over 9.5   E. None of these
        C. Between 6.0 and 7.0

154.   IODINE IS SOLUBLE IN WATER IN THE PRESENCE OF:
        A. Sodium citrate   D. PVP
        B. Sodium sulfate   E. PEG
        C. Lactose

155.   THE MOST SUCCESSFUL SULFONAMIDES HAVE WHAT TYPE OF SUB-
        STITUTION ON THE AMIDO NITROGEN:
        A. Carboxylic   D. Electronegative
        B. Alicyclic   E. Aliphatic
        C. Electropositive

156.   CHOLESTYRAMINE (QUESTRAN) CAUSES A NUMBER OF DRUG INTER-
        ACTIONS BECAUSE IT IS:
        A. Very acid in pH   D. Very alkaline in pH
        B. A complexing agent   E. Carrier substance
        C. A solubilizer

157.   POVAN COULD BE CLASSIFIED AS:
        A. A deflocculant   D. A disintegrator
        B. A lubricant   E. A surfactant
        C. A cyanine dye

158.   ALOES HAVE BEEN USED RECENTLY TO TREAT:
        A. Burns   D. Carcinomas
        B. Gastritis   E. Vertigo
        C. Blood dyscrasias

159. THE CLASS OF SUBSTANCES RESPONSIBLE FOR MOST ACCIDENTAL
      POISONINGS IN CHILDREN ARE:
      A. Detergents   D. Belladonna alkaloids
      B. Salicylate analgesics   E. Commercial dyes
      C. Bleaches

160. WHICH OF THE FOLLOWING CAN CAUSE DISCOLORATION OF TEETH?
      A. Chloromycetin   D. Kanamycin
      B. Penicillin   E. Sulfadiazine
      C. Achromycin

161. _____ CAN INCREASE THE SERUM LEVELS OF PENICILLINS
      SIGNIFICANTLY.
      A. Salicylates   D. Kaolin
      B. Probenicid   E. Starches
      C. Antacids

162. WHICH OF THE FOLLOWING SUBSTANCES IS NOT FOUND IN EMPIRIN
      COMPOUND TABLETS?
      A. Phenacetin
      B. Aspirin
      C. Diluent
      D. Acetanilid
      E. Lubricating agent

163. THE PRINCIPAL LIMITING FACTOR IN THE RATE OF ADSORPTION
      FROM SUSPENSIONS IS _____.
      A. Dissolution rate   D. Chemical stability
      B. Viscosity   E. Physical stability
      C. The suspending agent

164. PHENOBARBITAL ELIXIR CONTAINS IN EACH 100 CC. _____ GM.
      PHENOBARBITAL:
      A. 4.0   D. 0.1
      B. 1.0   E. 0.4
      C. 10.0

165. ULTRASONIC WAVES HAVE A FREQUENCY OF:
      A. 10-20 KC   D. Over 100 KC
      B. 20 KC or above   E. 80-90 KC
      C. 50 KC or above

      MATCH THE FOLLOWING:

166. ___ Gentamicin   A. Keflin
167. ___ Cephalexin   B. Nebs
168. ___ Ampicillin   C. Garamycin
169. ___ Fluocinamide   D. Totacillin
170. ___ Acetaminophen   E. Lidex

171. WHICH OF THE FOLLOWING SOLUTIONS SHOULD BE STERILE WHEN
      DISPENSED?
      A. Tinctures   D. Syrups
      B. Ophthalmic solutions   E. None of these
      C. Spirits

172. FILM COATINGS ARE:
      A. Enteric coatings   D. Very flexible
      B. Sustained release   E. Very thick
      C. Very brittle

173. A TYPE OF BOND FREQUENTLY SEEN IN COMPLEXES IS:
      A. Hydrogen bond   D. Double bond
      B. Ionic bond   E. Triple bond
      C. Semi-polar bond

174. AN EXAMPLE OF A UNIT DOSE INJECTABLE IS:
      A. Insulin
      B. Spersoids
      C. Tubex
      D. Spansule
      E. Clipsule

175. RADIOACTIVE DECAY FOLLOWS:
      A. A mixed order rate   D. A first order rate
      B. A fractional order rate   E. A second order rate
      C. A zero order rate

176. THE HLB SYSTEM IS USED TO CLASSIFY:
      A. Flavors   D. Organic ring structures
      B. Colors   E. Perfumes
      C. Surfactants

177. IN SITU SALT FORMATION USUALLY OCCURS:
      A. During in vivo distribution
      B. Before absorption
      C. In storage sites
      D. After biotransformation
      E. In the kidney

178. PASSIVE DIFFUSION:
      A. Can operate against a concentration gradient
      B. Is usually slow
      C. Requires high energy
      D. Is usually quite fast
      E. Requires low energy

179. IN ORDER TO MAKE AN ISO-ELIXIR CONTAINING 45% ALCOHOL,
      WHAT RATIO OF LOW 10% ISO-ELIXIR AND HIGH 75% ISO-ELIXIR
      SHOULD BE USED?
      A. 15 parts of 10% and 5 parts of 75%
      B. 6 parts of 10% and 7 parts of 75%
      C. 1 part of 10% and 6 parts of 75%
      D. 3 parts of 10% and 8 parts of 75%
      E. 5 parts of 10% and 3 parts of 75%

180.   RECTAL SUPPOSITORIES USUALLY WEIGH:
    A. 5 grams   D. 10 grams
    B. 2 grams   E. Vary in weight
    C. 1 gram

181.   OSTWALD PIPETTES ARE USED TO MEASURE:
    A. Specific gravity
    B. Samples for assay
    C. Density
    D. Osmotic pressure
    E. Viscosity

182.   ALPHA PARTICLES ARE VERY SIMILAR TO:
    A. Hydrogen atoms
    B. Helium atoms
    C. Neutrons
    D. Protons
    E. Electrons

183.   GAMMA RAYS ARE VERY SIMILAR TO:
    A. X-rays   D. Neutrinos
    B. Alpha radiation   E. Anti-neutrinos
    C. Beta radiation

184.   WHAT EFFECT DOES PLASMA PROTEIN BINDING HAVE ON ELIMINA-
    TION OF DRUGS?
    A. Slows it down
    B. Speeds it up
    C. Has no effect
    D. Changes the route of elimination
    E. Increases the proportion of metabolites

185.   A DRUG THAT REVERSES PLASMA PROTEIN BINDING IS OFTEN RE-
    FERRED TO AS:
    A. A protein hydrolysate   D. A carrier substance
    B. A displacer   E. An enzyme
    C. A solvate

186.   AN AVOIRDUPOIS POUND WEIGHS:
    A. 5,760 grains   D. 438 grains
    B. 454 grains   E. 480 grains
    C. 7,000 grains

187.   A RICH SOURCE OF VITAMIN A IS:
    A. Lean meats   D. Poultry
    B. Bread   E. Fish liver oils
    C. Liver

188.   CONTACT ANGLE IS USED TO MEASURE:
    A. Moisture content of granules
    B. Spreadability of ointments
    C. Disintegration of tablets
    D. Coefficient of friction of powders
    E. None of the above

189.   ACCORDING TO STOKES LAW, THE CREAMING OF EMULSIONS IS
        INDIRECTLY PROPORTIONAL TO:
        A. Density of the dispersed phase   D. Viscosity of the medium
        B. Gravity   E. None of these
        C. Radius of dispersed phase

190.   THE PERCENTAGE OF WATER IN LIQUEFIED PHENOL IS:
        A. 5%   D. 12. 5%
        B. 10%   E. 1%
        C. 15%

191.   THE MOST COMMON DISINTEGRATOR IN COMPRESSED TABLETS IS:
        A. Dextrose   D. Potassium bitartrate
        B. Lactose   E. Powdered sucrose
        C. Starch

192.   FREONS ARE:
        A. Alkanes   D. Fluorinated hydrocarbons
        B. Alkenes   E. Mixtures of CO_2 and air
        C. Alkynes

193.   AGGLOMERATION OF PARTICLES IN EMULSIONS IS OFTEN CALLED:
        A. Grouping
        B. Coalescence
        C. Dimerization
        D. Polymerization
        E. Dichromatism

194.   WHICH IS APPLICABLE TO ASCORBIC ACID?
        A. Deliquescent
        B. Absorbs CO2
        C. Oxidizes and yields a toxic compound
        D. Photosensitive
        E. None of these

195.   ABSORPTION OF VITAMIN A FROM THE GI TRACT DEPENDS ON:
        A. The presence of bile in the intestine
        B. Which salt is used
        C. Acid-base balance
        D. Needs of the patient
        E. pH of the intestine

196.   PURITY RUBRIC MEANS:
        A. Purified coloring substance
        B. Pure food and drug act
        C. U.S.P. or N.F. statement of required purity
        D. Substance requires purification
        E. None of these

197. WHICH OF THE FOLLOWING DOES NOT ENHANCE COMPLEXATION?
     A. Gums
     B. Cellulose derivatives
     C. Polyols
     D. Non-ionic surfactants
     E. Quaternary ammonium compounds

198. WHICH OF THE FOLLOWING FACTORS MAY MAKE IT NECESSARY TO
     GIVE LOWER DOSES OF DRUGS TO GERIATRIC PATIENTS?
     A. Reduction of enzyme activity   D. A and B
     B. Reduced kidney function   E. A, B and C
     C. Enhanced absorption

199. A DRUG THAT IS FREQUENTLY ADMINISTERED BY INHALATION IS:
     A. Insulin
     B. Isoproterenol
     C. Allopurinol
     D. Penicillin
     E. Nitroglycerin

200. A SOLUTION OF A VOLATILE SUBSTANCE IN ALCOHOL TO WHICH
     WATER IS SOMETIMES ADDED IS CALLED A(AN):
     A. Tincture
     B. Spirit
     C. Fluid extract
     D. Water
     E. Elixir

201. METHOTREXATE SHOULD NEVER BE USED CONCURRENTLY WITH:
     A. Penicillin
     B. Meprobamate
     C. Epinephrine
     D. Ethinamate
     E. Aspirin

202. TABLET HARDNESS RANGE IS NORMALLY:
     A. 0.2 - 0.5 Kg
     B. 0.5 - 1.0 Kg
     C. 1.0 - 2.0 Kg
     D. 2.0 - 3.5 Kg
     E. 3.5 - 7.0 Kg

203. AN ANTIDOTE FOR HEPARIN OVERDOSAGE IS:
     A. Protamine sulfate
     B. BAL
     C. Atropine
     D. Calcium salts
     E. Dicumarol

MATCH THE FOLLOWING POISONS WITH THE PROPER ANTIDOTE:

204. ___ Barium sulfide   A. BAL
205. ___ Arsenic   B. O_2 + CO_2
206. ___ Hydrocyanic acid   C. Ammonia water
207. ___ Formaldehyde   D. Epsom salts
208. ___ Iodine   E. Sodium formaldehyde sulfoxylate
209. ___ Opium   F. Calcium chloride
210. ___ Croton oil   G. Amyl nitrite
211. ___ Mercury bichloride   H. Starch
212. ___ Oxalic acid   I. Nalline
213. ___ Carbon monoxide   J. None of these

214. ANTICOAGULANT ACID CITRATE DEXTROSE INJECTION IS REQUIRED
      TO BE PYROGEN FREE. PYROGENS ARE:
      A. Organic catalysts formed in living cells
      B. Antigens contained in bacteria
      C. Non-specific globulins
      D. Products which stimulate hematopoietic organs
      E. Products causing febrile reaction upon injection

215. WEAKLY BASIC DRUGS ARE ELIMINATED BEST UNDER WHAT
      CONDITIONS?
      A. Alkaline urine   D. Slowed biotransformation
      B. Acid urine   E. Lack of biotransformation
      C. Neutral urine

216. ORAL HYPOGLYCEMICS ARE USUALLY MOST USEFUL IN:
      A. Juvenile diabetes   D. Late-onset diabetes
      B. Labile diabetes   E. Uncomplicated diabetes
      C. Brittle diabetes

217. ALCOHOL IS A SPECIFIC POTENTIATING AGENT WHEN USED WITH:
      A. Allopurinol   D. Sulfonamides
      B. Antihistaminics   E. Aspirin
      C. Penicillins

218. AMYL NITRITE IS USUALLY ADMINISTERED:
      A. By inhalation   D. I. V.
      B. Sublingually   E. Rectally
      C. I. M.

WHAT IS THE AVERAGE ORAL DOSE OF EACH OF THE
FOLLOWING?

219. ___ Povan   A. 5 mg/Kg
220. ___ Indocin   B. 100 mg
221. ___ Dexamethasone   C. 25 mg
222. ___ Erythromycin   D. 0.75 mg
223. ___ Dilantin   E. 250 mg

224. CAPSICUM IS USED IN O-T-C LINIMENTS TO:
    A. Promote easy spreading
    B. For its odor
    C. Produce warmth or heat
    D. As an analgesic
    E. None of the above

225. ALUMINUM CHLORIDE IS USED MAINLY AS A(AN):
    A. Antiemetic
    B. Laxative
    C. Suspending agent
    D. Urinary acidifier
    E. Antiperspirant

226. A SUBSTANCE THAT IS OFTEN USED TO SUBCOAT TABLETS IS:
    A. Sugar
    B. Carnauba wax
    C. Shellac
    D. Sodium stearate
    E. Sodium chloride

227. PENICILLIN G IS:
    A. Not used extensively in therapy
    B. The same as procaine penicillin
    C. The same as penicillin V
    D. Acid-stable
    E. Acid-labile

228. WHEN PRESCRIBING ORAL CONTRACEPTIVES, A PHYSICIAN NEED NOT GIVE SPECIAL ATTENTION TO WOMEN WHO HAVE:
    A. Migraine headaches   D. Never had a pregnancy
    B. Diabetes   E. High blood pressure
    C. Uterine tumors

MATCH THE FOLLOWING GENERIC NAMES WITH THE PROPER TRADE NAME:

229. ___ Mefanemic acid   A. Suavitil
230. ___ Chloromerodrin   B. Indocin
231. ___ Benactyzine   C. Placidyl
232. ___ Phenylbutazone   D. Neohydrin
233. ___ Chlorpromazine   E. Brevital
234. ___ Methohexital   F. Valmid
235. ___ Indomethacin   G. Butazolidin
236. ___ Ethchlorvynol   H. Thorazine
237. ___ Ethinamate   I. Ponstel
238. ___ Diphenidol   J. Vontrol

MATCH THE FOLLOWING:

239. ___ Methyl salicylate
240. ___ Sodium thiosulfate
241. ___ Iodides
242. ___ Ichthammol
243. ___ Hydrogen peroxide
244. ___ Nitrates
245. ___ Resorcinol
246. ___ Citrates
247. ___ Magnesium salts
248. ___ Phenol

A. Precipitated by alkali hydroxides
B. Solutions turn pink on exposure to air
C. Incompatible with ethyl nitrite
D. Broken down by heat, light, agitation
E. Should not be triturated with sugar
F. Acid solutions precipitate sulfur
G. Produces quinone with H_2O_2
H. Incompatible with vanishing cream
I. Forms insoluble calcium salts
J. Forms dark sticky mass with acidic
   substances

249. ETHER U. S. P. IS:
   A. Nonflammable
   B. Nonvolatile
   C. Water soluble
   D. Diethyl ether
   E. Dimethyl ether

250. A VITAMIN WHICH HAS SIGNIFICANT DEODORANT PROPERTIES IS:
   A. C
   B. A
   C. D
   D. E
   E. K

251. ANTABUSE IS USED TO TREAT:
   A. Diabetes
   B. Cholera
   C. Alcoholism
   D. Trench mouth
   E. Mumps

252. PHENTOLAMINE IS USED TO DIAGNOSE:
   A. Kidney function
   B. Ulcers
   C. Agranulocytosis
   D. Pheochromocytoma
   E. Mononucleosis

MATCH EACH DRUG WITH THE APPROPRIATE CAUTION TO THE PATIENT:

253. ___ Diphenylhydantoin
254. ___ Azogantrisin
255. ___ Povan
256. ___ Sinutabs
257. ___ Indocin

A. Stains the stool (red)
B. Stains the urine (red)
C. Take with coffee
D. Massage the gums
E. Take with solid food

258. WHICH OF THE FOLLOWING IS AVAILABLE IN A METERED DOSE AEROSOL?
   A. Reserpine
   B. Isoproterenol
   C. Guanethidine
   D. Dimenhydramine
   E. Diphenylhydantoin

259. WHICH OF THE FOLLOWING IS A NON-BARBITURATE GENERAL
     ANESTHETIC?
     A. Benzocaine
     B. Lidocaine (Xylocaine)
     C. Thiopental (Pentothal)
     D. Ketamine (Ketaject)
     E. None of the above

260. ADJUSTMENT OF DOSAGE OF DIPHENYLHYDANTOIN IS BASED
     PRIMARILY ON:
     A. Patient response   D. Body weight
     B. Blood levels   E. Prothrombin time
     C. Rate of excretion

261. DARVON-N CONTAINS_____ OF DEXTROPROPOXYPHENE
     NAPSYLATE.
     A. 50 mg   D. 65 mg
     B. 100 mg   E. None of these
     C. 32 mg

262. EPINEPHRINE (1:100) IS USUALLY ADMINISTERED:
     A. I. V.
     B. By inhalation
     C. I. M.
     D. Sub-lingually
     E. Not at all

263. WHICH OF THE FOLLOWING IS CONTRAINDICATED WITH MAO
     INHIBITORS?
     A. Milk   D. Meats
     B. Cheeses   E. Fish
     C. Cola beverages

     MATCH THE FOLLOWING:

264. ___ Marezine   A. Chloral hydrate
265. ___ Declomycin   B. Demethylchlortetracycline
266. ___ Noctec   C. Cyclizine
267. ___ Biphetamine   D. Amphetamine
268. ___ Ortho-Novum   E. Norethindrone

269. WHICH OF THE FOLLOWING IS NOT AN ADVANTAGE OF
     AEROSOL DOSE FORMS?
     A. Fine particle size   D. Even application
     B. Easy to apply   E. Less contamination
     C. Inexpensive

270. WHICH OF THE FOLLOWING MAY BE USED AS PLASMA EXPANDERS?
     A. Sodium salts
     B. Dextrans
     C. Starches
     D. Calcium salts
     E. Prostaglandins

271. WHICH IS ADDED TO GLYCERIN PREPARATIONS TO MINIMIZE
THE IRON TANNIN DISCOLORATION?
A. Exsiccated sodium sulfite and sodium citrate
B. Disodium hydrogen phosphate
C. Citric acid and sodium citrate
D. Sodium bisulfite
E. Sodium dihydrogen phosphate

272. RED DYE NO. 3 WAS BANNED BY FDA BECAUSE OF POSSIBILITY OF
INCREASED INCIDENCE OF:
A. Stability problems   D. Impurities
B. Carcinomas   E. Allergic reactions
C. Kidney problems

273. A PRESCRIPTION CALLS FOR 500 MG OF DIGOXIN DISSOLVED IN
ENOUGH SOLVENT TO MAKE 3 FLUID OUNCES. HOW MUCH OF
THIS SOLUTION WILL CONTAIN APPROXIMATELY 1/30 GR. OF
DIGOXIN?
A. 5 minims   D. 10 minims
B. 4 minims   E. 6 minims
C. 8 minims

274. WHICH OF THE FOLLOWING IS OFTEN USED AS A HUMECTANT?
A. Glycerin   D. Tween 20
B. Sodium chloride   E. None of these
C. Ethanol

275. MOST BINDERS USED IN TABLETING ARE:
A. Gums   D. Starches
B. Waxes   E. Clays
C. Oleoresins

MATCH THE FOLLOWING DRUGS WITH THEIR SOURCES:

276. ___ Insulin   A. The earth
277. ___ Penicillin G   B. Animal pancreas
278. ___ Kaolin   C. Molds
279. ___ Chondrus   D. Sea moss
280. ___ Cantharides   E. Insects

281. AN ANTIEMETIC THAT CONTAINS MAINLY CARBOHYDRATE
DERIVATIVES IS:
A. Vesprin   D. Thorazine
B. Compazine   E. Emetrol
C. Tigan

282. _____ IS USED TO OFFSET THE EFFECTS OF COUMARIN
DERIVATIVES.
A. Protamine sulfate
B. Adrenalin
C. Vitamin K
D. Calcium
E. BAL

283. ENSEALS ARE A TRADEMARK DOSE FORM NAME OF:
    A. Abbott   D. Ciba
    B. Lilly   E. Pfizer
    C. Parke Davis

284. THE USUAL RESULT OF TRITURATING CAMPHOR AND MENTHOL
    TOGETHER IS A (AN):
    A. Synergistic effect
    B. Antagonistic effect
    C. Hydrotropic solvent
    D. Eutectic mixture
    E. Compound solution

285. MOST VOLATILE OILS ARE RICH IN:
    A. Terpenes   D. Gluco-corticoids
    B. Sulfur containing compounds   E. Pyrimidines
    C. Fluorinated hydrocarbons

286. WHICH ONE OF THE FOLLOWING IS TRUE CONCERNING METHADONE
    HCl?
    A. Dissolves in water with the aid of sodium bicarbonate
    B. Its solutions undergo rapid hydrolysis
    C. Its solutions can be sterilized by autoclaving
    D. Stabilized by addition of sodium bicarbonate
    E. Precipitates from aqueous solutions by alcohol

    MATCH THE FOLLOWING:

287. ___ Novobiocin   A. Quite insoluble in water and organic
288. ___ Nystatin   solvents, soluble in aqueous alcohols
289. ___ Sodium penicillin G   B. Calcium salt more stable in aqueous
290. ___ Chloramphenicol palmitate   solution than sodium salt
291. ___ Neomycin sulfate   C. Extremely stable and active in
                               alkaline solutions
                         D. Inactivated by alcohol
                         E. Must be hydrolyzed in intestines to
                               be active

292. THE MAXIMUM NUMBER OF REFILLS FOR A DRUG COVERED BY THE
    DRUG ABUSE ACT IS:
    A. 5   D. 3
    B. 1   E. p. r. n.
    C. 6

293. THE FIRST NON-SEDATIVE DRUG USED TO TREAT EPILEPSY WAS:
    A. Ethotoin   D. Mysoline
    B. Tridione   E. Diphenylhydantoin
    C. Paradione

293. WHICH OF THE FOLLOWING STATISTICAL TECHNIQUES IS (ARE) USE-
    FUL FOR CLINICAL TRIALS?
    A. F Test
    B. Chi Square Test
    C. Latin Square
    D. A and B above
    E. All of the above

294. WHICH OF THE FOLLOWING IS NOT USED AS A BINDER
     FOR TABLETS?
     A. Talc   D. Sucrose
     B. Starch   E. Gelatin
     C. Glucose

     MATCH THE FOLLOWING:

295. ___ Kaolin and pectin   A. Nembutal
296. ___ Trimethadione   B. Kaopectate
297. ___ Pentobarbital   C. Selsun
298. ___ Selenium sulfide   D. Neosynephrine
299. ___ Phenylephrine   E. Tridione

300. ___ Tetrex   A. Analgesic
301. ___ Elavil   B. Anthelminthic
302. ___ Povan   C. Antibiotic
303. ___ Ananase   D. Tranquilizer
304. ___ Zactirin   E. Anti-inflammatory agent

305. GMP REGULATIONS (U.S.F.D.A.) APPLY PRIMARILY TO:
     A. Controlled drugs   D. Hospital pharmacy
     B. Wholesalers   E. Community pharmacy
     C. Pharmaceutical manufacturers

306. pH IS EQUIVALENT TO pKa AT:
     A. pH of 7   D. Half neutralization point
     B. pH of 1   E. Neutralization point
     C. pH of 14

307. CAUSATIVE PARASITES OF MALARIA BELONG TO THE GENUS:
     A. Plasmodium   D. Shigella
     B. Mycobacterium   E. Streptomyces
     C. Pasteurella

308. A METHOD FOR REMOVING PYROGENS FROM WATER INVOLVES:
     A. Oxidation with permanganate
     B. Oxidation with H_2O_2
     C. Precipitation with H_2S
     D. Absorption on certain asbestos filter pads
     E. None of the above

309. SPLITTING OFF OF THE FACE OF A TABLET IS CALLED:
     A. Capping   D. Whiskering
     B. Fissuring   E. Picking
     C. Slugging

310. AN INSTRUMENT USED TO MEASURE DURABILITY OF TABLETS
     TO SHOCK AND ABRASION IS A:
     A. Tensiometer   D. Brittleometer
     B. Dart penetrometer   E. Friabilator
     C. Chilsonator

311.   THE DUPONT TRADE NAME FOR FLUORINATED HYDROCARBONS IS:
    A. Isotrons   D. Ucons
    B. Genetrons   E. None of these
    C. Freons

312.   THE NON-AQUEOUS VEHICLE USED IN INJECTIONS IS:
    A. Alcohol
    B. Glycerol
    C. Alcoholic sodium stearate
    D. Vegetable oils
    E. Wax or liquid petrolatum

313.   MEDICAL LETTER IS PRIMARILY DEVOTED TO:
    A. Updates in laws
    B. Drug evaluations
    C. Editorials
    D. Drug interactions
    E. None of the above

MATCH EACH OF THE FOLLOWING DRUGS WITH THE APPROPRIATE
DESCRIPTIONS:

314. ___ Butazolidin   A. Blue and white capsule
315. ___ Achromycin V   B. Green and black capsule
316. ___ Darvon Comp. 65   C. Red coated tablet
317. ___ Indocin   D. Red capsule
318. ___ Donnazyme   E. Blue and yellow capsule
319. ___ Librium 10 mg   F. Oval pink tablet
320. ___ Miradon   G. Red and gray capsule
321. ___ Dexedrine   H. Green coated tablet
322. ___ Noctec   I. Green and yellow layered
323. ___ Norgesic   tablet
                                J. Triangular orange tablet

324.   MICROMERITICS IS:
    A. The science of small particles
    B. A microscopic blood count method
    C. A method of chemical analysis
    D. An optical instrument
    E. Colorimetry

325.   MOST TESTS OF STATISTICAL SIGNIFICANCE ARE BASED ON THE:
    A. Null hypothesis
    B. Mean
    C. Standard deviation
    D. Range
    E. Chi Square test

326. INFATABS (P. D.) HAVE THE FOLLOWING SHAPE:
    A. Ovoid   D. Triangular
    B. Round   E. Oblong
    C. Four-leaf clover

327. MERCURIC CHLORIDE:
    A. Corrodes surgical instruments
    B. Is not bacteriostatic
    C. Is extremely toxic
    D. Is called calomel
    E. Is insoluble in water

MATCH THE FOLLOWING:

328. ___ Penicillin G   A. Allylmercaptomethylpenicillin
329. ___ Penicillin O   B. Phenoxymethylpenicillin
330. ___ Penicillin V   C. Benzylpenicillin

331. THE EQUATION FOR A STRAIGHT LINE IS A = MX + B. M REPRESENTS:
    A. The initial value of x
    B. The slope of the line
    C. The intercept with the y axis
    D. The intercept with the x axis
    E. The initial value of y

332. THE BOILING POINT OF ALCOHOL IS 78° C. THE CORRESPONDING TEMPERATURE IN DEGREES FARENHEIT IS:
    A. 46   D. 156
    B. 110   E. 140
    C. 172

333. FOR OPHTHALMIC USE, BORIC ACID SOLUTION SHOULD BE:
    A. Diluted with an equal volume of distilled water
    B. Undiluted
    C. Diluted with an equal volume of isotonic saline solution
    D. Diluted with an equal volume of sterile distilled water
    E. Diluted with an equal volume of sterile isotonic saline solution

334. WHICH OF THE FOLLOWING MAY STAIN THE BODY AND CLOTHING?
    A. Meprobamate   D. Kaopectate
    B. Benadryl   E. Acidulin
    C. Povan

335. BORIC ACID IS MORE SOLUBLE IN:
    A. Glycerin than water
    B. Water than glycerin
    C. Water than in boiling water
    D. Alcohol than in glycerin
    E. Alcohol than in boiling water

336. A PHYSICIAN WRITES A PRESCRIPTION THAT REQUIRES 3/4 GRAIN
      OF AMPHETAMINE. HOW MANY 5 MG. TABLETS SHOULD THE
      PHARMACIST USE TO FILL THE PRESCRIPTION?
      A. 9 1/2   D. 9 3/4
      B. 11   E. 7 1/2
      C. 8

337. IN STOKES' LAW:
      A. Rate of settling is directly proportional to particle diameter
      B. Viscosity is directly proportional to particle diameter
      C. Temperature is important
      D. Conc. of suspended phase is unimportant
      E. None of these

338. A POPULAR THEORY OF ACIDS AND BASES IS:
      A. Boyle's Law
      B. 4 Humors' Theory
      C. Pythagorean Theory
      D. Bronsted-Lowry Theory
      E. Henry's Theory

339. SALICYLIC ACID IS USED PRIMARILY AS A(AN):
      A. Analgesic   D. Uricosuric agent
      B. Antipyretic   E. Keratolytic agent
      C. Cough suppressant

340. POTASSIUM IODIDE IS FREQUENTLY USED AS A SATURATED SOLUTION
      WHOSE STRENGTH w/v IS APPROXIMATELY:
      A. 0. 9%   D. 15. 5%
      B. 50%   E. 100%
      C. 70%

341. PRESERVED WATER IS MADE BY ADDING_____TO PURI-
      FIED WATER:
      A. Phenol   D. Parabens
      B. Benzoic acid   E. None of these
      C. Zephiran

342. WHICH OF THE FOLLOWING ACIDS IS NORMALLY FOUND IN THE
      LIQUID STATE IN NATURE?
      A. Lactic acid   D. Barbituric acid
      B. Tartaric acid   E. Salicylic acid
      C. Benzoic acid

343. WHICH OF THE FOLLOWING IS AN EXPECTORANT AGENT?
      A. Codeine
      B. Dextromethorphan
      C. Glyceryl guaiacolate
      D. Glycerin
      E. Wild cherry syrup

344. A PRIMARY DISADVANTAGE OF COOL AIR VAPORIZERS IS:
    A. Discomfort
    B. Noise
    C. Staining properties
    D. Lack of effectiveness
    E. No automatic shut-off

345. VEEGUM IS:
    A. A polyol
    B. An organic gum
    C. A synthetic gum
    D. A clay
    E. A non-ionic surfactant

346. THE USUAL PERCENTAGE OF ACTIVE DRUG IN FLUID EXTRACTS IS:
    A. 1%
    B. 10%
    C. 20%
    D. 90%
    E. 100%

347. A DISADVANTAGE OF CHLORAL HYDRATE IS:
    A. Lack of absorption
    B. Rapid elimination
    C. Lack of chemical stability
    D. Causes allergic reactions
    E. Disagreeable odor

348. A COMMON CONTAMINANT OF ETHER U. S. P. IS:
    A. Ethanol
    B. Methanol
    C. Ketones
    D. Peroxides
    E. Heavy metals

349. GLYCERIN IS EMPLOYED IN IPECAC SYRUP BECAUSE IT:
    A. Insures more perfect solubility of ipecac
    B. Minimizes hydrolysis of tannins
    C. Prevents precipitation of tannins
    D. Acts as fungicide
    E. None of these

350. THE CROCKER-HENDERSON SYSTEM IS USED TO CLASSIFY:
    A. Flavors
    B. Dyes
    C. Odors
    D. Surfactants
    E. Deflocculants

351. EPSOM SALT WHEN EXPOSED TO AIR IS:
    A. Deliquescent
    B. Anhydrous
    C. Hygroscopic
    D. Efflorescent
    E. None of these

MATCH THE FOLLOWING SUBSTANCES WITH THE FUNCTIONS THEY SERVE:

352. ___ Sodium citrate in tannic acid glycerite   A. Prevents discoloration
353. ___ Methylparaben in hydrophilic ointment   B. To form soap
354. ___ Magnesium oxide in aromatic cascara   C. Retards extraction of bitter
      sagrada fluid extract   principals
355. ___ Sodium borate in cold cream   D. Preservative
356. ___ Alcohol in medicinal soft soap liniment   E. Solubilizes active ingredient
357. ___ Hydrochloric acid in nux vomica tr.   F. Vehicle

358. A SOLID OR SEMISOLID FATTY MEDICINAL PREPARATION INTENDED FOR EXTERNAL USE AND WHICH SOFTENS OR MELTS AT BODY TEMPERATURE IS CALLED:
     A. Glycerite   D. Ointment
     B. Gel   E. Emulsion
     C. Mucilage

359. AN AQUEOUS SOLUTION OF ALUMINUM CHLORIDE IS:
     A. Neutral   D. Amphoteric
     B. Acid   E. None of these
     C. Alkaline

MATCH THE FOLLOWING:

360. ___ Monsel's solution   A. Ammoniacal silver nitrate solution
361. ___ Dobell's solution   B. Sulfurated lime lotion
362. ___ Vleminckx's solution   C. Ammonium acetate solution
363. ___ Spirit of Mindererus   D. Aluminum acetate solution
364. ___ Lead water   E. Ferric subsulfate solution
365. ___ Howe's solution   F. Lead subacetate solution
366. ___ Burow's solution   G. Diluted lead subacetate solution
367. ___ Goulard's extract   H. Sodium borate solution

MATCH THE FOLLOWING:

368. ___ Atabrine   A. Dramamine
369. ___ Dimenhydrinate   B. Rolicton
370. ___ Glyceryl Triacetate   C. Quinacrine
371. ___ Isoproterenol   D. Enzactin
372. ___ Amisometradine   E. Isuprel

373. PYRVINIUM PAMOATE (POVAN) DOSAGE IS USUALLY ADJUSTED ACCORDING TO:
     A. Age
     B. Biological half-life
     C. Prothrombin time
     D. Physiological state
     E. Body weight

374. WHICH OF THE FOLLOWING IS CONTAINED IN A NUMBER OF SUN
     TANNING LOTIONS?
     A. Benzocaine   D. Benzoic acid
     B. PABA   E. Salicylic acid
     C. Zinc oxide

     MATCH THE USUAL ADULT DOSE WITH THE DRUG TO WHICH IT
     APPLIES:

375. ___ Librium   A. 1/150 gr. stat.
376. ___ Declomycin   B. 10 mg. t. i. d.
377. ___ Tripelennamine   C. 50 mg. q. 4 h.
378. ___ Meprobamate   D. 150 mg. q. i. d.
379. ___ Glyceryl trinitrate   E. 400 mg. q. i. d.

380. A TYPE OF FLOW IN WHICH VISCOSITY INCREASES WHEN THE
     SUBSTANCE IS AGITATED IS:
     A. Newtonian   D. Plastic
     B. Dilatant   E. Thixotropic
     C. Pseudoplastic

381. LENTE INSULIN IS:
     A. Only given intravenously
     B. 70% crystalline, 30% amorphous insulin
     C. 30% crystalline, 70% amorphous insulin
     D. Another name for NPH insulin
     E. The shortest acting insulin preparation

     MATCH THE FOLLOWING:

382. ___ Erythromycin   A. Soluble in water, suitable
383. ___ Erythromycin ethyl carbonate   for I. V. use
384. ___ Erythromycin glucoheptonate B. Acidic solutions rapidly
                                         deteriorate
                                      C. Useful for extemporaneous
                                         preparations

     MATCH THE FOLLOWING:

385. ___ Alphaprodine   A. Perin
386. ___ Dextropropoxyphene   B. Diaparene
387. ___ Dextromethorphan   C. Darvon
388. ___ Methylbenzethonium chloride D. Romilar
389. ___ Piperazine calcium edathamil E. Nisentil

390. AMISOMETRADINE IS:
     A. A carbonic anhydrase inhibitor
     B. A mercurial diuretic
     C. A non-mercurial diuretic
     D. A uricosuric agent
     E. None of these

391. PROBENECID SHOULD NOT BE USED IN THE TREATMENT OF GOUT IN
      CONJUNCTION WITH SALICYLATES BECAUSE:
      A. The toxicity of probenecid is increased by the acidic salicylates
      B. Probenecid is not effective in gout
      C. Therapeutic actions are antagonistic
      D. Their actions are synergistic
      E. None of these

MATCH THE FOLLOWING:

392. ___ Trimeprazine   A. Vioform
393. ___ Glutethimide   B. Doriden
394. ___ Ethinamate   C. Terramycin
395. ___ Iodochlorhydroxyquin   D. Valmid
396. ___ Chlordiazepoxide   E. Placidyl
397. ___ Ethchlorvynol   F. Temaril
398. ___ Oxytetracycline   G. Librium

399. THE USUAL CONCENTRATION OF KCL IN HYPERALIMENTATION FLUIDS
      IS _____ PER L.
      A. 1 Gm   D. 4 m Eq.
      B. 2 Gm   E. 40 m Eq.
      C. 1 m Eq.

MATCH THE FOLLOWING:

400. ___ Long release tablet   A. Medihaler
401. ___ Sublingual tablet   B. Glosset
402. ___ Aerosol device   C. Abboject
403. ___ Color flecked tablet   D. Gradumet
404. ___ Disposable syringe   E. Medilet

405. IPSATOL CONTAINS _____ AS AN EXPECTORANT.
      A. Ammonium chloride
      B. Ipecac
      C. Glyceryl guaiacolate
      D. Potassium iodide
      E. None of the above

406. ALL TETRACYCLINE ANTIBIOTICS:
      A. Have the same chemical structures but are stereoisomers
      B. Are destroyed by alkali hydroxides
      C. Produce the same incidence of side effects
      D. Are isolated from streptococcus rinosus
      E. All are true

407. DIHYDROSTREPTOMYCIN:
      A. Is more effective than streptomycin
      B. Is less toxic than streptomycin
      C. Is isolated from a bacillus
      D. Must not be injected I.V.
      E. None of these

408. AQUEOUS SUSPENSIONS OF _____ MAY BE KEPT AT ROOM
TEMPERATURE FOR 3 WEEKS WITHOUT SIGNIFICANT LOSS OF
POTENCY.
   A. Sodium penicillin G
   B. Chloroprocaine penicillin O
   C. Penicillin G
   D. Penicillin V
   E. Penicillin O

409. THE CONCENTRATION OF NITROFURAZONE SOLUTIONS USED
OPHTHALMICALLY IS:
   A. 2%   D. 5%
   B. 20%   E. 1%
   C. 0.02%

410. DMSO IS NO LONGER USED CLINICALLY BECAUSE IT WAS
FOUND TO PRODUCE:
   A. Agranulocytosis   D. Eye damage
   B. Skin damage   E. Carcinomas
   C. Brain damage

411. THE IDEAL ANTISEPTIC CONCENTRATION OF ETHYL
ALCOHOL IS:
   A. 95%   D. 50%
   B. 70%   E. 75%
   C. 100%

412. _____ IS NOT METABOLIZED BY THE LIVER.
   A. Phenobarbital   D. Allobarbital
   B. Barbital   E. Secobarbital
   C. Pentobarbital

MATCH THE FOLLOWING:

413. ___ Methadone   A. Povan
414. ___ Mephobarbital   B. Mebaral
415. ___ Conjugated estrogens   C. Premarin
416. ___ Pyrinium pamoate   D. Dolophine
417. ___ Dimenhydrinate   E. Dramamine

418. RISTOCETIN:
   A. Is isolated from a strain of bacillus
   B. Is well absorbed orally
   C. Can only be given intravenously
   D. Preferable route of administration is I.M.
   E. Is a single chemical entity

419. PYRIDOXINE IS:
   A. Vitamin B6
   B. Vitamin A
   C. Vitamin B1
   D. Vitamin K
   E. Vitamin D

44   SECTION I - PHARMACY

MATCH THE FOLLOWING:

420. ___   Pyribenzamine   A. Anti-epileptic
421. ___   Dilantin   B. Diuretic
422. ___   Meprobamate   C. Tranquilizer
423. ___   Diamox   D. Sedative
424. ___   Tuinal   E. Antihistamine

425. ___   Carbomycin   A. Magnamycin
426. ___   Cycloserine   B. Spontin
427. ___   Erythromycin   C. Sumycin
428. ___   Ristocetin   D. Ilotycin
429. ___   Tetracycline phosphate E. Seromycin

430. WHICH OF THE FOLLOWING IS THE MOST EFFECTIVE SUN SCREEN?
      A. PABA
      B. Titanium dioxide
      C. Methoxysoralen
      D. Menthyl salicylate
      E. Baby oil

MATCH THE FOLLOWING:

431. ___   Contac   A. Multiple vitamin
432. ___   Maalox   B. Cough syrup
433. ___   Formula 44   C. Poison ivy therapy
434. ___   Dramamine   D. Diarrhea control
435. ___   Caligesic   E. Motion sickness
436. ___   Unicap   F. Hemorrhoids
437. ___   Kaopectate   G. Antacid
438. ___   Glycerin suppositories H. Antiseptic
439. ___   Anusol   I. Cold therapy
440. ___   Merthiolate   J. Laxative

441. A DISADVANTAGE OF SACCHARIN IS:
      A. Bitter aftertaste
      B. Lack of solubility
      C. Low degree of sweetness
      D. Lack of stability in solution
      E. None of the above

442. TUINAL (LILLY) CONTAINS AMOBARBITAL AND:
      A. Pentobarbital   D. Aspirin
      B. Phenobarbital   E. Caffeine
      C. Secobarbital

443. GLYCERINATED GELATIN IS A(AN):
      A. Suspension   D. Emulsion
      B. Solid   E. None of these
      C. Colloidal solution

444. WHAT IMPARTS THE PINK COLOR TO CALAMINE?
    A. Zinc oxide   D. Carmine
    B. Titanium dioxide   E. F.D.C. Red #3
    C. Ferric oxide

MATCH THE FOLLOWING:

445. ___ Emollient	A.	Stimulates perspiration
446. ___ Diaphoretic	B.	Increases R.B.C. count
447. ___ Febrifuge	C.	Evacuates gall bladder
448. ___ Cholegogue	D.	Softens skin
449. ___ Vermifuge	E.	Decreases body temperature
450. ___ Hematopoietic	F.	Kills worms

MATCH THE FOLLOWING:

451. ___ Dextropropoxyphene	A.	Zactane
452. ___ Micronized griseofulvin	B.	Declomycin
453. ___ Penicillin G	C.	Pentids
454. ___ Ethoheptazine	D.	Fulvicin V
455. ___ Penicillin O	E.	Darvon
456. ___ Demethylchlortetracycline	F.	Cer-O-Cillin
457. ___ Prednisolone	G.	Thorazine
458. ___ Tripelennamine	H.	Pyribenzamine
459. ___ Meprobamate	I.	Meticortelone
460. ___ Chlorpromazine	J.	Tetrex
461. ___ Dihydromorphinone	K.	Equanil
462. ___ Tetracycline	L.	Dilaudid

WHAT IS THE CORRECT SOURCE OF THE FOLLOWING DRUGS?

463. ___ Agar	A.	Gadus morrhua
464. ___ Gentian	B.	Red algae
465. ___ Benzoin	C.	Resin from bark
466. ___ Dried stomach	D.	Secretion of apis mellifera
467. ___ Theelin	E.	Rhizomes and roots
468. ___ Cod liver oil	F.	Urine of pregnant mares
469. ___ Rabies vaccine	G.	Killed fixed virus from rabbit brain
470. ___ Yellow wax	H.	Goa powder
471. ___ Wool fat	I.	Sheep
472. ___ Chrysarobin	J.	Hog

473. GLYCERIN HAS A SPECIFIC GRAVITY OF 1.25. ONE GALLON WEIGHS:
    A. 591.25 grams   D. 128 grams
    B. 473 grams   E. 4800 grams
    C. 4730 grams

MATCH THE FOLLOWING:

474. _C_ 1 fluid dram   A. 64. 8 mg.
475. ___ 1 pint   B. 128 fluid ounces
476. ___ 1 milliliter   C. 60 min.
477. ___ 1 grain   D. 60 grains
478. ___ 1 gallon   E. 473 ml.
479. ___ 1 apothecary dram   F. 16. 23 min.
                                     G. None of these

480. ONE APOTHECARY OUNCE EQUALS:
      A. 480 grains   D. 473 grains
      B. 28. 35 grains   E. None of these
      C. 29. 57 grains

481. ONE AVOIRDUPOIS OUNCE IS EQUIVALENT TO:
      A. 480 grains   D. 15. 432 grains
      B. 437. 5 grains   E. None of these
      C. 454. 6 grains

482. ONE AVOIRDUPOIS OUNCE EQUALS:
      A. 454. 6 grams   D. 28. 35 grams
      B. 31. 1 grams   E. None of these
      C. 29. 57 grams

483. ONE APOTHECARY OUNCE EQUALS:
      A. 16 grams   D. 28. 35 grams
      B. 31. 1 grams   E. None of these
      C. 29. 57 grams

484. ONE FLUID OUNCE EQUALS:
      A. 15 ml.   D. 29. 57 ml.
      B. 3. 69 ml.   E. None of these
      C. 28. 35 ml.

485. ONE FLUID OUNCE EQUALS:
      A. 480 min.   D. 128 min.
      B. 15. 432 min.   E. None of these
      C. 454. 6 min.

486. ONE GRAM EQUALS:
      A. 16. 23 grains
      B. 31. 1 grains
      C. 15. 432 grains
      D. 16 grains
      E. None of these

MATCH THE TRADEMARK DOSE NAME WITH THE APPROPRIATE
COMPANY:

487. _E_ Mistometer   A. Schering
488. _G_ Kapseals   B. Lilly
489. _B_ Gelseals   C. Ciba-Geigy
490. _C_ Linguets   D. Lederle
491. ___ Dulcets   E. ~~Winthrop~~
492. _H_ Tabule   F. ~~S. K. F.~~
493. _A_ Medilets   G. ~~Parke-Davis~~
494. _D_ Sequels   H. Neisler
495. _C_ Spacetabs   I. Upjohn
496. _F_ Spansule   J. Abbott
497. ___ Medules   K. Ayerst
498. _L_ Secule   L. ~~Sandoz~~

MATCH THE FOLLOWING:

499. _A_ Salt   A. $RCOONa$
500. _C_ Ester   B. $RCOCl$
501. ___ Acid anhydride   C. ~~$RCOOC_2H_5$~~
502. ___ Acyl halide   D. ~~$RCONH_2$~~
503. _D_ Acyl amide   E. $(RCO)_2O$

MATCH THE FOLLOWING PREPARATIONS WITH THE PROPER
LABELLING OR STORAGE DIRECTIONS:

504. ___ Smallpox vaccine   A. Poison label
505. ___ Mild silver protein solution   B. None of these
506. ___ Burow's solution   C. External use only
507. ___ Strong ammonia solution   D. Store below 0° C
508. ___ Liver solution   E. Solutions should not be
         applied over long periods
         of time
         F. Light-resistant container

MATCH EACH OF THE FOLLOWING DRUGS WITH ITS PRIMARY
THERAPEUTIC CLASS:

509. ___ Meperidine   A. Anti-epileptic
510. ___ Secobarbital   B. Antifungal
511. ___ Mephenesin   C. Sedative
512. ___ Tolnaftate   D. Hormone
513. ___ Lidocaine   E. Narcotic analgesic
514. ___ Ethotoin   F. Cough suppressant
515. ___ Testosterone   G. Muscle relaxant
516. ___ Dextromethorphan   H. Local anesthetic
517. ___ Probenecid   I. Anti-arthritic
518. ___ Methotrexate   J. Anti-carcinoma

MATCH THE CORRECT INGREDIENT WITH THE FOLLOWING
PHARMACEUTICAL PREPARATIONS:

519. ___	Lugol's solution	A.	Hydrochloric acid
520. ___	Desenex	B.	Chlortrimeton
521. ___	Acidulin	C.	Boric acid
522. ___	Ziradryl	D.	Iodine
523. ___	Benylin expectorant	E.	Pectin
524. ___	Collyrium	F.	Zinc undecylenate
525. ___	Coricidin	G.	Zirconium salt
526. ___	Kaopectate	H.	Glyceryl guaiacolate
527. ___	Formula 44 Cough syrup	I.	Albamycin
528. ___	Panalba	J.	Cetamium

529. TINCTURES:
A. Are made by direct solution of a volatile oil
B. Represent 100 gm. of drug to 100 ml. of finished tincture
C. Are aqueous solutions of active constituents of drugs
D. Are sweetened, flavored aqueous alcoholic solutions of drugs
E. Are none of these

530. VITAMIN K IS ASSOCIATED WITH:
A. Pellagra
B. Nerves
C. Hemoglobin concentration
D. Bones
E. Blood clotting

531. WHICH IS FOUND IN VITAMIN B_{12}?
A. Magnesium
B. Nickel
C. Iron
D. Cobalt
E. Manganese

MATCH THE FOLLOWING:

532. A Excipient
533. E Oleoresin
534. C Marc
535. B Syrup
536. D Nebula

A. An inert adhesive or adsorbent
   substance used in making pill masses
B. Aqueous solution of sucrose
C. Residue from extraction of a drug
D. A solution of a drug in light liquid
   petrolatum
E. None of these

MATCH THE FOLLOWING:

537. C Levigation
538. D Calcination
539. B Trituration
540. E Exsiccation
541. A Contusion

A. Crushing of a drug by bruising and
   pounding
B. Grinding of a substance to a very
   fine powder
C. Process of finely powdering an
   inorganic substance by rubbing it
   with a liquid in which it is insoluble
D. Heating inorganic substance to drive
   off volatile constituents
E. Removal of all water from a substance with strong heat

MATCH THE FOLLOWING:

542.	A	Comminution	A. Reduction of particle size
543.	D	Ebullition	B. Roasting
544.	B	Torrefaction	C. Vaporization
545.	C	Sublimation	D. Boiling
546.	G	Colation	E. Percolation
547.	H	Expression	F. Method of extraction
548.	E	Lixiviation	G. Straining
549.	F	Maceration	H. Forcible separation of liquids from
550.	J	Lyophilization	solids
551.	I	Emulsion	I. Dispersion of an oil in water
			J. Freeze drying

MATCH THE FOLLOWING:

552. ___	Indocin	A. Anti-malarial
553. ___	Doriden	B. Diuretic
554. ___	Talwin	C. Analgesic
555. ___	Larodopa	D. Anti-neoplastic agent
556. ___	Velban	E. Anti-arthritic
557. ___	Vontrol	F. Anti-migraine therapy
558. ___	Plaquenil	G. Hypnotic
559. ___	Sansert	H. Hypoglycemic agent
560. ___	Edecrin	I. Anti-emetic
561. ___	Dymelor	J. Parkinson's syndrome

MATCH THE FOLLOWING:

562. ___	Antipyretic	A. Benzyl benzoate
563. ___	Emulsifier	B. Tolbutamide
564. ___	Treatment of scabies	C. Acetanilid
565. ___	Anti-malarial	D. Quinine
566. ___	Hypoglycemic agent	E. Sodium lauryl sulfate
567. ___	Analgesic	F. Probantheline
568. ___	Anti-spasmodic	G. Ethoheptazine
569. ___	Anti-fungal	H. Griseofulvin

MATCH THE FOLLOWING:

570. ___	Talwin	A. Antihistaminic
571. ___	Temaril	B. Migraine therapy
572. ___	Indocin	C. Cough preparation
573. ___	Tensilon	D. Vaginal antifungal
574. ___	Quelidrine	E. Muscle relaxant
575. ___	Benadryl	F. Non-narcotic analgesic
576. ___	Compazine syrup	G. Anti-pruritic
577. ___	Robaxin	H. Anti-arthritic
578. ___	Sansert	I. Anti-emetic
579. ___	Tridione	J. Mood elevator
580. ___	Naqua	K. Diagnostic for myasthenia gravis
581. ___	Elavil	L. Diuretic
582. ___	Hyva	M. Anticonvulsant

MATCH EACH OF THE OTC DRUGS WITH ITS PROPER CLASS:

583. ___ Kao-Con		A.	External analgesic
584. ___ Sominex		B.	Eye wash
585. ___ Cheracol		C.	Anti-diarrheal
586. ___ Metrecal		D.	Sleep aid
587. ___ Orajel		E.	Internal analgesic
588. ___ Riopan		F.	Toothache remedy
589. ___ Musterole		G.	Cough preparation
590. ___ Solarcaine		H.	Diet food
591. ___ Preparation H		I.	Burn remedy
592. ___ Collyrium		J.	Laxative
593. ___ Ziradryl		K.	Treat hemorrhoids
594. ___ Kondremul		L.	Antacid
595. ___ Tempra		M.	Poison ivy remedy

596. ANOTHER NAME FOR POLYETHYLENE GLYCOL POLYMERS IS:
     A. Sodium alginate   D. Friar paste
     B. Silica gel   E. None of these
     C. Carbowax

597. P. E. G. 400 MONOSTEARATE IS NOT MISCIBLE WITH:
     A. Water   D. Benzene
     B. Alcohol   E. Isopropyl alcohol
     C. Ether

MATCH THE FOLLOWING:

598. ___ Col.		A.	Every hour
599. ___ Coch. mag.		B.	According to the art
600. ___ Pulv.		C.	Let be swallowed
601. ___ Omn. hor.		D.	Mix
602. ___ S. A.		E.	Carbonated water
603. ___ Ft.		F.	Strain
604. ___ M.		G.	A powder
605. ___ Deglut.		H.	A large spoonful
606. ___ Si op. sit		I.	A drop
607. ___ Ag. aeratq.		J.	Make
608. ___ Ut dict.		K.	Dust or sprinkle
609. ___ Gtt.		L.	If necessary
610. ___ Stat.		M.	As directed
611. ___ Consperg.		N.	Immediately

MATCH THE ABBREVIATIONS IN COLUMN I, WITH THE CORRECT
STATEMENT IN COLUMN II:

612. ___	O. S.	A. If necessary
613. ___	q. i. d. a. c. et h. s.	B. Left eye
614. ___	pro re nata	C. A teaspoonful
615. ___	si opus sit	D. Every other day
616. ___	coch. parv.	E. 4 times a day before meals and at
617. ___	O. U.	bedtime
618. ___	d. t. d. no. IV	F. Both eyes
619. ___	dieb. alt.	G. Give four such doses
620. ___	e. m. p.	H. Let a gargle be made
621. ___	fiat. garg.	I. As directed
		J. When necessary

MATCH THE FOLLOWING OTC DRUGS WITH THEIR PRINICIPAL ACTIVE
INGREDIENT :

622. ___	Listerine	A. Sulfur
623. ___	Jayne's PW	B. Benzocaine
624. ___	Robitussin	C. Phenylmercuric nitrate
625. ___	Poli-Grip	D. Iodochlorhydroxyquin
626. ___	Solarcaine	E. Glyceryl guaiacolate
627. ___	Preparation H	F. Gentian violet
628. ___	Acnomel	G. Karaya gum
629. ___	Vioform Powder	H. Salicylic acid
630. ___	Panscol Lotion	I. Hexylresorcinol

631. THE HYDROGEN ION CONCENTRATION OF A SOLUTION WITH A pH OF
5. 6 IS:

A. 3.9×10^{-5}　　　　　D. 7.0×10^{-5}
B. 2.5×10^{-6}　　　　　E. 7.0×10^{-6}
C. 2.5×10^{-5}

632. AN OPHTHALMIC PREPARATION SHOULD HAVE A pH OF _____
TO CONFORM TO THAT OF LACRIMAL FLUID.

A. 6.2-6.8　　　　　D. 9.2-10
B. 7.2-8.0　　　　　E. None of these
C. 8.4-9.0

MATCH THE FOLLOWING:

633. ___	Zinc undecylenate	A. Paradione
634. ___	Paramethadione	B. Coumadin
635. ___	Pipamazine	C. Compazine
636. ___	Warfarin	D. Desenex
637. ___	Phenindione	E. Fungizone
638. ___	Prochlorperazine	F. Mornidine
639. ___	Amphotericin B	G. Neutrapen
640. ___	Sulfisoxazole	H. Serpasil
641. ___	Penicillinase	I. Hedulin
642. ___	Reserpine	J. Polycillin
643. ___	Ampicillin	K. Gantrisin
644. ___	Norethynodrel	L. Enovid

645.   HOW MANY ML. OF A 5% STOCK SOLUTION SHOULD BE USED TO
        PREPARE 4 FLUID OUNCES OF A 1:200 SOLUTION?
        A. 48 ml.
        B. 10 ml.
        C. 4 ml.
        D. 1. 2 ml.
        E. 12 ml.

646.   SEQUENTIAL ORAL CONTRACEPTIVES ARE USED FOR _____
        TOTAL DAYS OF THE CYCLE.
        A. 20 or 21   D. 10 or 11
        B. 16   E. 28
        C. 18 or 19

647.   A SOLUTION IS PREPARED BY DISSOLVING A ONE OUNCE PACKAGE
        OF DRUG IN ONE FLUIDOUNCE OF WATER. WHAT IS THE % W/W OF
        THE RESULTING SOLUTION?
        A. 100%   D. 46. 5%
        B. 50%   E. 33. 3%
        C. 48. 6%

648.   THE ADULT DOSE OF A DRUG IS 250 MG. WHAT DOSE SHOULD BE
        GIVEN TO A 9 MONTH-OLD BABY ACCORDING TO FRIED'S RULE?
        A. 15 mg.   D. 9 mg.
        B. 0. 15 Gm.   E. 0. 0025 Gm.
        C. 3/8 gr.

649.   -12° C. IS EQUIVALENT TO_____°F.
        A. 36   D. 5
        B. 12   E. -2
        C. 10. 4

650.   2 DRACHMS IS EQUIVALENT TO_____Gm.
        A. 8. 0   D. 2. 6
        B. 3. 0   E. None of these
        C. 4. 1

651.   ONE TABLESPOONFUL IS APPROXIMATELY EQUIVALENT TO
        _____ML.
        A. 15   D. 20
        B. 10   E. 30
        C. 8

MATCH THE FOLLOWING:

652.	A	Doxycycline	A. Vibramycin
653.	B	Pancrelipase	B. Cotazym
654.	M	Methacycline	C. Banthine
655.	I	Carbamazepine	D. Hygroton
656.	O	Diazepam	E. Betalin
657.	G	Metaxolone	F. Doriden
658.	C	Methantheline	G. Skelaxin
659.	N	Nitrofurazone	H. Compazine
660.	J	Phenindione	I. Tegretol
661.	H	Prochloroperazine	J. Hedulin
662.	F	Glutethimide	K. Ilotycin
663.	E	Thiamine	L. Thorazine
664.	K	Erythromycin	M. Rondomycin
665.	D	Chlorthalidone	N. Furacin
666.	E	Vitamin B_1	O. Valium

MATCH THE FOLLOWING:

667.	E	Desoxyn	A. Ayerst
668.	I	Talwin	B. Schering
669.	B	Grisactin	C. Ciba
670.	J	Orinase	D. Lilly
671.	C	Serpasil	E. Warner-Lambert
672.	I	Miltown	F. Abbott
673.	B	Chlortrimeton	G. Winthrop
674.	D	Darvon	H. Roche
675.	D	V Cillin K	I. Wallace
676.	H	Librium	J. Upjohn

MATCH THE FOLLOWING:

677.	G	Auralgan	A. Winthrop
678.	E	Dilantin	B. Parke-Davis
679.	A	Grifulvin	C. MSD
680.	E	Selsun	D. Wyeth
681.	I	Pentids	E. Roche
682.	D	Unipen	F. Abbott
683.	E	Gantrisin	G. Ayerst
684.	J	Pan-Alba	H. McNeil
685.	A	Aralen	I. Squibb
686.	C	Aldomet	J. Upjohn

687.   IN STREPTOCOCCAL INFECTIONS, PENICILLINS SHOULD BE CON-
TINUED FOR:
A. 15 days
B. 10 days
C. a week
D. 5 days
E. 3 days

688. N.A.B.P. REGULATIONS REQUIRE AT LEAST _____ HOURS
OF INTERNSHIP TRAINING FOR LICENSURE AS A PHARMACIST.
A. 400
B. 1500
C. 2000
D. 750
E. 1000

689. MOST DIARRHEA REMEDIES CONTAIN:
A. Kaolin
B. Benzocaine
C. Aluminum oxide
D. Paregoric
E. Citric acid or citrates

690. ANOTHER NAME FOR METHADONE IS:
A. Aminomone
B. Dionin
C. Metaphenone
D. Dolophine
E. Dolamine

691. SYRUP U.S.P. CONTAINS_____% (W/V) OF SUCROSE.
A. 35
B. 40
C. 50
D. 65
E. 85

692. DISCLOSING SOLUTIONS ARE USED TO:
A. Stain plaque
B. Act as abrasives
C. Dissolve food particles
D. Wash away food debris
E. Sterilize the oral cavity

693. WHICH IS NOT A NATURAL ALKALOID:
A. Ergotamine
B. Scopolamine
C. Papaverine
D. Lobeline
E. Apomorphine

694. CALAMINE CONTAINS:
A. Al_2O_3
B. CaO
C. ZnO
D. FeO
E. $CaCO_3$

695. IRRADIATION OF ERGOSTEROL YIELDS:
A. Cholesterol
B. Eugenol
C. Ergotoxine
D. Calciferol
E. Ergonovine

696. ACNOMEL IS USUALLY USED TO TREAT:
A. Burns
B. Hemorrhoids
C. Diarrhea
D. Indigestion
E. Acne

697. A TEST SOLUTION FOR ALKALOIDS USED TO TEST FOR COMPLETE-
NESS OF EXTRACTION:
A. Silver nitrate
B. Gold chloride
C. Mercury potassium iodide
D. Mercuric oxide
E. Hydrogen sulfide

698. THE PRINCIPAL CONSTITUENT OF OIL OF PEPPERMINT IS:
    A. Citrol   D. Menthol
    B. Cineol   E. Carvone
    C. Eugenol

699. WHICH STATEMENT CORRECTLY DESCRIBES THE SOLUBILITY OF
    ALKALOIDS?
    A. Sparingly soluble in water, soluble in dilute acid
    B. Sparingly soluble in water, soluble in non-polar solvent
    C. Sparingly soluble in water, insoluble in dilute acid
    D. Insoluble in water, insoluble in dilute acid
    E. Insoluble in water, insoluble in non-polar solvent

700. BARRIER CREAMS ARE QUITE USEFUL IN PREVENTING:
    A. Drug allergies   D. Psoriasis
    B. Poison sumac   E. Dry skin
    C. Food allergies

701. STABILIZER IN MAGNESIA MAGMA:
    A. Benzoic acid   D. Lactic acid
    B. Citric acid   E. Mandelic acid
    C. Oxalic acid

702. THE ACTIVE INGREDIENT OF DESENEX SOLUTION IS:
    A. Salicylic acid   D. Basic fuchsin
    B. Glyceryl triacetate   E. None of these
    C. Undecylenic acid

703. ENZACTIN RELEASES _____ IN THE PRESENCE OF
    FUNGUS:
    A. Undecylenic acid
    B. Salicylic acid
    C. Acetic acid
    D. Nitric acid
    E. Hydrochloric acid

704. TINACTIN CONTAINS THE ANTIFUNGAL:
    A. Tolnaftate   D. Undecylenic acid
    B. Glyceryl triacetate   E. None of these
    C. Zinc undecylenate

705. A SUSTAINED RELEASE DOSAGE FORM THAT RELEASES DRUG
    FROM A PLASTIC MATRIX IS:
    A. Spacetabs   D. Strasionic products
    B. Gradumets   E. Emplets
    C. Spansule

706. WOOL WAX ALCOHOL IS:
    A. Cholesterol
    B. Cetyl alcohol
    C. Stearyl alcohol
    D. Myricyl alcohol
    E. Phytosterol

707.	STABILIZER PERMITTED IN AMINOPHYLLIN INJECTION:
	A. Urea					D. Nicotinamide
	B. Thioglycolic acid			E. Ethylenediamine
	C. Quinine and urea

708.	SERUTAN IS CLASSIFIED AS A (AN) _____ LAXATIVE.
	A. Saline					D. Bulk Forming
	B. Emollient				E. None of these
	C. Stimulant

709.	THE CHIEF USE OF VEEGUM IS:
	A. Surfactant				D. Anti-oxidant
	B. Suspending agent			E. Preservative
	C. Deflocculant

710.	MIDOL IS USED MAINLY FOR:
	A. Menstrual cramps			D. Athlete's foot
	B. Headache				E. Psoriasis
	C. Arthritic pain

711.	WHICH OF THE FOLLOWING SHOULD BE CLASSIFIED AS A
	DEFLOCCULATING AGENT?
	A. Tween 20				D. Sodium lauryl sulfate
	B. Marasperse				E. Carbowax
	C. Tween 80

712.	SELSUN BLUE IS USED MAINLY AS A (AN):
	A. Skin lotion				D. Ointment
	B. Shampoo				E. Aerosol
	C. Bath additive

713.	PAREGORIC CONTAINS 4% BY VOLUME OF OPIUM TINCTURE. HOW
	MANY MG. OF MORPHINE ARE CONTAINED IN ONE DESSERTSPOON-
	FUL OF PAREGORIC?
	A. 16					D. 32
	B. 4					E. 3.2
	C. 8

714.	TELEPHONED PRESCRIPTIONS ARE PERMITTED UNDER DEA
	REGULATIONS FOR SCHEDULES:
	A. II through V				D. I through V
	B. IV and V				E. None of these
	C. III through V

715.	INSULIN INJECTION MAY BE DISTINGUISHED FROM PROTAMINE ZINC
	INJECTION AS:
	A. Insulin injection is more viscous owing to its higher glycerin content
	B. Protamine zinc insulin contains no phenol odor
	C. Protamine zinc insulin is colorless while insulin injection is yellowish
	D. Insulin injection is acid to litmus while protamine is not
	E. Protamine zinc insulin injection is a white suspension while insulin
	    injection is a clear fluid

716. A-200 PYRINATE IS USED MAINLY:
   A. To kill lice
   B. To treat pinworms
   C. To treat tapeworm
   D. To treat fungus infections
   E. None of these

717. CARBOWAX COMPOUNDS MAY BE CLASSIFIED AS:
   A. Isomers
   B. Tautomers
   C. Polymers
   D. Epimers
   E. None of these

MATCH THE FOLLOWING:

718. ___ An aerosol propellant
719. ___ A gum
720. ___ A cyanine dye
721. ___ A carbohydrate mixture
722. ___ A viscosimeter
723. ___ A balance
724. ___ A colorimeter
725. ___ A tablet hardness tester
726. ___ A blender
727. ___ A mill

A. Ainsworth
B. DuBosc
C. Strong-Cobb
D. Stormer
E. Povan
F. Acacia
G. Emetrol
H. Patterson-Kelly
I. Fitz
J. Freon 11

728. MENTHOL IS CLASSIFIED AS A (AN):
   A. Open chain terpene alcohol
   B. Monocyclic terpene alcohol
   C. Dicyclic terpene alcohol
   D. Aromatic phenol
   E. Heterocyclic alcohol

729. THE PRINCIPAL OXIDATION PRODUCT OF ETHYLENE GLYCOL IS:
   A. Ethanol
   B. Citric acid
   C. Carbon monoxide
   D. Oxalic acid
   E. Acetaldehyde

730. MOST DEPILATORIES CONTAIN:
   A. Thioglycollates
   B. Bismuth salts
   C. Sulfur
   D. Salicylic acid
   E. Formates

731. THE AMOUNT OF 190 PROOF REQUIRED TO MAKE 500 CC. OF 70%
   ALCOHOL IS:
   A. 350
   B. 520
   C. 184
   D. 368
   E. 37

732. ANTIPERSPIRANTS FREQUENTLY CONTAIN:
   A. Ammonium salts
   B. Undecylenates
   C. Zinc salts
   D. Sulfonate salts
   E. Aluminum salts

733. WHICH ONE OF THE FOLLOWING IS INSOLUBLE IN ALCOHOL?
      A. Resins   D. Ether
      B. Esters   E. Gums
      C. Volatile oils

734. WHAT IS THE pH OF A SOLUTION WHICH HAS A HYDROXYL ION CON-
      CENTRATION OF 1.0×10^{-11}?
      A. 10   D. 3
      B. 4   E. 11
      C. 2

MATCH THE FOLLOWING:

735. ___ Continental method   A. Rheology
736. ___ Granulation   B. Buffers
737. ___ Freezing point depression method C. Tableting
738. ___ Van Slyke equation   D. Isotonic solutions
739. ___ Newtonian   E. Emulsions

WHAT WOULD YOU DISPENSE FOR THE FOLLOWING DRUGS?

740. ___ Diphenhydramine   A. Aureomycin
741. ___ Chlorpromazine   B. Benadryl
742. ___ Procaine   C. Gantrisin
743. ___ Norepinephrine   D. Acthar gel
744. ___ N-allylnormorphine   E. Nalline
745. ___ Chlortetracycline   F. Novocaine
746. ___ Sulfisoxazole   G. Pyribenzamine
747. ___ Tripelennamine   H. Demerol
748. ___ Adrenocorticotrophic hormone   I. Thorazine
749. ___ Meperidine HCl   J. Levarterenol

750. MANY OTC CORN REMEDIES CONTAIN:
      A. Undecylenic acid   D. Bichloracetic acid
      B. Nitric acid   E. Salicylic acid
      C. Trichloracetic acid

751. BETADINE CONTAINS:
      A. Benzocaine   D. Gentian violet
      B. Surfacaine   E. Beta-methionine
      C. Povidone-iodine complex

752. WHICH OF THE FOLLOWING DOSE FORMS IS SPECIFICALLY COVERED
      BY THE FEDERAL "HAZARDOUS SUBSTANCES LABELING ACT"?
      A. Parenterals   D. Ophthalmic solutions
      B. Aerosols   E. Nitroglycerin tablets
      C. Tinctures

753. THE U.S.P. SPECIFICATION OF A "COOL PLACE" INCLUDES THE
      RANGE:
      A. 8 to 15°C
      B. 0 to 10°C
      C. 0 to 20°C
      D. -5 to +5°C
      E. None of the above

754. HOW MANY CC. OF 1:1000 EPINEPHRINE SOLUTION ARE NECESSARY TO
MAKE 30 CC. OF A 1:5000 SOLUTION?
A. 10 cc.   D. 60 cc.
B. 6 cc.   E. 8 cc.
C. 4 cc.

755. BCG IS USUALLY ADMINISTERED:
A. S.C. in small frequent doses   D. S.C. in 2 divided doses
B. I.M. in single dose   E. S.C. on alternate days (3
C. Intradermally in a single dose   doses)

756. BACID IS USED MAINLY TO TREAT:
A. Gastritis   D. Diarrhea
B. Infections   E. Indigestion
C. Constipation

757. A LONG-ACTING GLYCOSIDE OF DIGITALIS IS:
A. Digoxin   D. Digitalin
B. Gitalin   E. Digitoxin
C. Digora

758. BENZOCAINE IS MOST EFFECTIVE TOPICALLY IN CONCENTRATIONS
OF:
A. 20%   D. 1%
B. 5%   E. 50%
C. 2%

759. SORBITOL IS USEFUL MAINLY AS A (AN):
A. Solubilizer   D. Counter-irritant
B. Surfactant   E. Humectant
C. Emulsifier

760. THE FOLLOWING IS A COMPONENT OF HYDROPHILIC OINTMENT AND
IS MAINLY RESPONSIBLE FOR ITS PROPERTIES:
A. Glycerin   D. Cetyl alcohol
B. Propyl paraben   E. Propylene glycol
C. Sodium lauryl sulfate

761. QUINTESS (LILLY) CONTAINS:
A. Cetylpyridinium   D. Kaolin
B. Activated attapulgite   E. Pectin
C. Kaolin, pectin

762. ESTROGENIC ACTIVITY OF PREMARIN IS EXPRESSED IN TERMS OF
CONTENT OF:
A. Estradiol benzoate
B. Estrone sulfate
C. Ethinyl benzoate
D. Theelin
E. Stilbesterol

763. SCOPOLAMINE IS FREQUENTLY USED IN OTC SLEEP AIDS AS THE
      _____ DERIVATIVE.
      A. HCl   D. Methionate
      B. Sulfate   E. Aminoxide HBr
      C. Phosphate

764. A GROUP OF SUBSTANCES USED AS SUPPOSITORY BASES THAT
      DISSOLVE RATHER THAN MELT ARE:
      A. Esters
      B. Saturated acids
      C. Carbowaxes
      D. Unsaturated fatty acids
      E. None of these

765. INDOCIN IS MARKETED BY:
      A. Lilly   D. Pfizer
      B. Squibb   E. Merck Sharpe & Dohme
      C. Upjohn

766. GLY-OXIDE IS USED FREQUENTLY TO TREAT:
      A. Hypoxia   D. Dental caries
      B. Trench mouth   E. Dyspepsia
      C. Worm infestations

767. THE OFFICIAL TITLE OF EPSOM SALT IS:
      A. Sodium bicarbonate   D. Sodium sulfate
      B. Alum   E. Potassium iodide
      C. Magnesium sulfate

768. RECIPROCITY OF PHARMACY LICENSURE IS PRIMARILY A
      FUNCTION OF:
      A. A. Ph. A.   D. A. I. H. P.
      B. A. A. C. P.   E. A. F. P. E.
      C. N. A. B. P.

769. RECORDS RELATING TO DEA DRUGS MUST BE PRESERVED FOR:
      A. 1 year   D. 7 years
      B. 2 years   E. Permanently
      C. 5 years

770. AN AGENT COMMONLY COMBINED WITH LOCAL ANESTHETICS IS:
      A. Epinephrine   D. Isoproterenol
      B. Phenylephrine   E. None of these
      C. Ephedrine

771. A PATIENT TAKING PYRIDIUM SHOULD BE WARNED ABOUT:
      A. Marked drowsiness
      B. Gastric distress
      C. Headaches
      D. Discoloration of the urine
      E. Dizziness

772. WHEN NON-POLAR SUBSTANCES ARE DISSOLVED IN A POLAR SOLVENT USING SURFACTANTS, THE PROCESS IS CALLED:
   A. HLB
   B. Solubilization
   C. Emulsification
   D. Gelatination
   E. None of these

773. POLYSORBATE IS A SYNONYM FOR:
   A. Spans
   B. Sodium lauryl sulfate
   C. Tweens
   D. Brij
   E. Stannous fluoride

774. DIPHENHYDRAMINE IS PRODUCED BY:
   A. Parke-Davis
   B. Lederle
   C. Merck Sharpe & Dohme
   D. Wyeth
   E. None of these

775. THE ANTIDOTE FOR DDT POISONING IS:
   A. Adrenalin
   B. Atropine
   C. Barbiturate
   D. Amphetamine
   E. Glycerol monoacetate

776. SELSUN IS INTENDED PRIMARILY FOR USE ON THE_____.
   A. Scalp
   B. Skin
   C. Hair
   D. Toes
   E. Feet

777. OXYCEL IS USED MAINLY AS A (AN):
   A. Thickener
   B. Emulsifier
   C. Oxidizing agent
   D. Hemostat
   E. Surfactant

778. TRANSFER OF DEA CONTROLLED DRUGS BETWEEN PHARMACIES HAS A _____% LIMIT.
   A. 5
   B. 10
   C. 1
   D. 2
   E. 6

779. CONTAC IS:
   A. A skin cream
   B. A cold preparation
   C. An aerosol
   D. A parenteral
   E. A barbiturate

780. WHICH OF THE FOLLOWING IS A CLASS I CONTROLLED DRUG:
   A. Paregoric
   B. Heroin
   C. Morphine
   D. Demerol
   E. None of the above

781.   THE CHEMICAL SUBSTANCE USED COMMONLY IN RUNNING A G. I.
       SERIES IS:
       A.   Barium sulfate
       B.   Fluorescein dye
       C.   Radioactive iodine
       D.   Sodium bicarbonate
       E.   Sodium carbonate

782.   COLLEGES OF PHARMACY ARE ACCREDITED BY:
       A.   A. F. P. E.
       B.   A. A. C. P.
       C.   A. C. P. E.
       D.   N. A. B. P.
       E.   None of the above

MATCH EACH PRODUCT WITH ITS PRINCIPAL USE:

       A.   Cold remedy
       B.   Analgesic
       C.   Athlete's foot remedy
       D.   Prickly heat
       E.   Dentifrice
       F.   Antacid

783.   _____ Aveeno
784.   _____ Calurin
785.   _____ Allerest
786.   _____ Tinactin
787.   _____ Neutrox
788.   _____ Amitone

MATCH THE FOLLOWING:

       A.   Riker
       B.   Abbott
       C.   Lederle
       D.   P. D.
       E.   Merrell

789.   _____ Infatab
790.   _____ Dospan
791.   _____ Spersoid
792.   _____ Gradumet
793.   _____ Medihaler

MATCH THE FOLLOWING DRUGS WITH THE MANUFACTURER:

A.   Purdue Frederick
B.   U. S. Vitamin
C.   Whitehall
D.   Rorer
E.   Lederle
F.   Davies, Rose-Hoyt
G.   Schering

794. C Dristan
795. E Orabase
796. B Aquasol A
797. A Betadine
798. F Rhulispray
799. D Carfusin
800. G Tinactin

FOR EACH OF THE FOLLOWING MULTIPLE CHOICE QUESTIONS, CHOOSE THE ONE MOST APPROPRIATE ANSWER:

801. THE EMETIC ACTION OF MORPHINE IS DUE TO:
  A. Irritation of gastrointestinal tract
  B. Stimulation of cerebral cortex
  C. Stimulation of medullary vomiting center
  D. Stimulation of emetic chemoreceptor trigger zone
  E. None of these

802. ONE SPECIFIC SIDE EFFECT OF TRIDIONE ADMINISTRATION IS:
  A. Severe gingival hyperplasia   D. Cerebral depressions
  B. The "glare phenomenon"   E. All of these
  C. Respiratory depression

803. COLCHICINE IS USED MAINLY TO TREAT:
  A. Gout   D. Carcinomas
  B. Arthritis   E. High blood pressure
  C. Diabetes

804. ONE PROCEDURE IN THE TREATMENT OF DIGITALIS POISONING IS TO:
  A. Give K^+ salts
  B. Reduce or stop the administration of the drug
  C. Administer quinidine
  D. Use permanganate or tannin chemical antidote
  E. Administer diuretics to the patient

805. THE ACTION OF QUINIDINE DIFFERS FROM THAT OF DIGITALIS IN:
  A. Decreasing irritability of cardiac muscle
  B. Preventing passage of impulses to the ventricle
  C. Increasing irritability of heart muscle
  D. Reducing conductivity
  E. None of the above

806. WHICH OF THE FOLLOWING WOULD BE CONTRAINDICATED DURING ANTABUSE THERAPY?
  A. Pentobarbital   D. Paradione
  B. Paraldehyde   E. None of these
  C. Chloral hydrate

807. _____ IS A DRUG ADMINISTERED BY INHALATION OF POWDER AS A PROPHYLACTIC FOR ASTHMA.
  A. Ephedrine   D. Oxytriphylline
  B. Disodium cromolyn   E. Epinephrine
  C. Isoproterenol

808. MORPHINE STIMULATES:
  A. Biliary and pancreatic secretions
  B. Non-propulsive rhythmic contractions of small intestine of man
  C. Propulsive contractions in small intestine of man
  D. Propulsive peristaltic waves in colon
  E. Human uterus at full term

MATCH THE DRUG WITH THE DISEASE IT IS MOST OFTEN USED FOR:

809. C Myleran   A. Hodgkin's disease
810. A Nitrogen mustard A   B. Chronic lymphatic leukemia
811. E Triethylenemelamine   C. Chronic myeloma
812. B Leukeran b   D. Multiple myeloma
813.   Urethane P   E. Acute lymphoblastic leukemia

MATCH THE FOLLOWING:

814. C Donnatol   A. Cardiac glycoside
815. B Ergonovine   B. Oxytoxic
816. E Sparine   C. Spasmolytic
817. D Tripelennamine   D. Antihistamine
818. A Ouabain   E. Ataractic

819. N-ACETYLCYSTINE IS CLASSIFIED AS A (AN):
      A. Analgesic
      B. Antitussive
      C. Mucolytic agent
      D. Antitubercular agent
      E. Protein hydrolysate

820. DRUGS USED TO TREAT CYSTIC FIBROSIS INCLUDE ALL EXCEPT:
      A. Anticholinergics   D. Expectorants
      B. Antibiotics   E. Pancreatic enzymes
      C. Mucolytic agents

821. BARBITURATES ARE METABOLIZED MAINLY IN THE:
      A. Stomach   D. Kidney
      B. Small intestine   E. Liver
      C. Spleen

822. OVER-USE OF DIGITALIS MAY RESULT IN:
      A. Habituation   D. Physical dependence
      B. Tolerance   E. Cumulative poisoning
      C. Addiction

MATCH THE FOLLOWING:

823. D Colchicine   A. Skeletal muscle relaxant
824. A Curare   B. Megaloblastic anemias
825.   Diamox   C. Used in hypertension
826. B Folic acid   D. Used in gout
827. C Serpasil   E. Non-mercurial diuretic

828. THE BRAIN STEM CENTERS AFFECTED MOST STRONGLY BY
      BARBITURATES ARE:
      A. The respiratory centers
      B. The vasomotor centers
      C. The cardioinhibitory centers
      D. The cardioacceleratory centers
      E. None of the above

15
20

829.   THE HYPNOTIC DOSE OF A BARBITURATE:
        A. Acts mainly on the cerebral cortex
        B. Acts primarily on the brain stem
        C. Acts primarily on the thalamus
        D. Has a general action on the entire central nervous system
        E. None of the above

830.   STRYCHNINE DEATHS IN HUMANS USUALLY OCCUR FROM:
        A. Cardiac failure
        B. Exhaustion of the respiratory center
        C. Fatigue of spinal reflexes
        D. Fatigue of respiratory muscles
        E. Kidney failure

        MATCH THE FOLLOWING:

831.   ___ Cafergot   A. Anti-inflammatory
832.   ___ Amyl nitrite   B. Shock
833.   ___ Levophed   C. Coronary dilator
834.   ___ Ananase   D. Anti-migraine
835.   ___ Tacaryl   E. Anti-histaminic

836.   STRYCHNINE ACTS BY:
        A. Stimulating acetylcholine production
        B. Stimulating nerve cell metabolism
        C. Depressing inhibitory centers in the spinal cord
        D. Inhibiting cholinesterase
        E. Stimulating production of cholinesterase

837.   THE FATAL BLOOD LEVEL OF ETHYL ALCOHOL IS APPROXIMATELY:
        A. 0.25 mg./vol.   D. 1.50 mg./vol.
        B. 0.75 mg./vol.   E. 5.00 mg./vol.
        C. 0.50 mg./vol.

838.   THE ACTION OF DIGITALIS IS ENHANCED BY:
        A. Sodium   D. Potassium
        B. Calcium   E. Chloride
        C. Magnesium

839.   WHICH OF THE FOLLOWING MAY PRECIPITATE AN ASTHMA ATTACK?
        A. Respiratory acidosis   D. Cranberry juice
        B. Viral and bacterial infections   E. Chocolate or coca cola
        C. Respiratory alkalosis

840.   DOSAGE OF ANTICONVULSANTS ARE ADJUSTED:
        A. When attacks occur frequently
        B. Every two weeks
        C. Every two years
        D. Only when side effects are seen
        E. Seasonally

841. THE FIRST TOXIC SYMPTOMS OF DIGITALIS POISONING ARE:
    A. Gastrointestinal irritation   D. Cerebral excitement
    B. Undue depression of heart rate   E. Colored vision
    C. Flushing of skin

842. ENZYMATIC OXIDATION OF TRAPPED IODIDES IS BLOCKED IN THE THYROID GLAND BY:
    A. Iodides   D. Penicillin
    B. Telepaque   E. Thyroxin
    C. Thiourea

843. A DRUG THAT PRODUCES INCREASED CONTRACTION OF THE SPHINCTER IRIDIS BY LOCAL APPLICATION IS A:
    A. Parasympathomimetic drug   D. Sympatholytic drug
    B. Parasympatholytic drug   E. None of the above
    C. Sympathomimetic drug

GIVE THE CHIEF USE OF EACH OF THE FOLLOWING:

844. _____ Naqua   A. Migraine headache
845. _____ Velban   B. Tranquilizer
846. _____ Librium   C. Diuretic
847. _____ Cafergot   D. Antihistaminic
848. _____ Equanil   E. Anti-carcinogenic
849. _____ Diuril
850. _____ Benadryl

MATCH THE FOLLOWING SIDE EFFECTS WITH THE DRUG PRODUCING THEM:

    A. Tinnitis
    B. Skin rashes
    C. Hypertrophy of the gums
    D. Discoloration of teeth

851. _____ Soma
852. _____ Dilantin
853. _____ Achromycin
854. _____ Streptomycin

SECTION II - PHARMACOLOGY

MATCH THE DRUG WITH THE MOST CORRECT ORAL ADULT DOSE:

855. C Pyribenzamine   A. 250 mg.
856. C Meperidine HCl   B. 15 mg.
857. A Chloraquine   C. 50 mg.
858. B Ephedrine HCl   D. 100 mg.
859. E Ergotamine   E. 0.5 mg.
860. A Chloramphenicol
861. D Papaverine HCl
862. E Colchicine

863. ALL BUT ONE OF THE FOLLOWING SYMPTOMS ARE PRESENT IN
     DIGITALIS INTOXICATION:
     A. A-V block
     B. Ventricular tachycardia
     C. Vomiting
     D. Vagal arrest of the heart
     E. Visual disturbances

864. TERBUTALINE HAS A PREFERENCE FOR STIMULATION OF _____
     RECEPTORS.
     A. Alpha   D. Beta 2
     B. Gamma   E. Dopaminergic
     C. Beta 1

865. BAL (BRITISH ANTI-LEWISITE) IS USED TO COUNTERACT THE TOXIC
     EFFECTS OF:
     A. Atropine   D. Barbiturates
     B. Mercury   E. Digitalis
     C. Morphine

866. STREPTOMYCIN CAN CAUSE:
     A. 4th cranial nerve damage   D. 6th cranial nerve damage
     B. 8th cranial nerve damage   E. Blindness
     C. 10th cranial nerve damage

867. CARBACHOL IS:
     A. Rapidly hydrolyzed by acetylcholinesterase
     B. Without nicotinic properties
     C. A potent muscarinic drug
     D. Administered in a dose of 5 to 10 mg. twice a day
     E. Enhanced in activity by prior administration of eserine

868. WHICH OF THE FOLLOWING SHOULD NOT BE ADMINISTERED TO A
     PATIENT WITH MYASTHENIA GRAVIS?
     A. Prostigmine   D. Curare
     B. Digitalis   E. Insulin
     C. Atropine

869. ALCOHOL IN THE BODY IS:
     A. Oxidized to CO_2 and water
     B. Excreted by lungs
     C. Excreted by kidneys
     D. Excreted by large intestine
     E. Detoxified by kidney

870. ASPIRIN DELAYS ABSORPTION OF:
      A. Tetracycline
      B. Digoxin
      C. Propranolol
      D. Indomethacin
      E. Penicillin

871. METHANOL MAY CAUSE:
      A. Deafness   D. Gastritis
      B. Tetany   E. Blindness
      C. Delirium tremens

872. THE TOXICITY OF METHANOL IS DUE TO ITS CONVERSION IN THE
      BODY TO:
      A. Acetaldehyde   D. Carbonic acid
      B. Formic acid and formaldehyde E. Methane
      C. Ethyl alcohol

873. AN UNDESIRABLE SIDE REACTION SOMETIMES SEEN WITH AMINO-
      PYRINE IS:
      A. Leukemia   D. Methemoglobinemia
      B. Sickle cell anemia   E. Mononucleosis
      C. Agranulocytosis

874. _____ MAY INCREASE THE INSULIN NEED OF DIABETICS.
      A. Isoniazid   D. Aspirin
      B. Penicillin   E. Prednisone
      C. Glyceryl guaiacolate

875. WHICH OF THE FOLLOWING IS NOT SIGNIFICANTLY ABSORBED ORALLY?
      A. Isoproterenol
      B. Cromolyn
      C. Ephedrine
      D. Cephalexin
      E. Theophylline

876. BECAUSE THE ACTION OF DICUMAROL PERSISTS FOR SEVERAL DAYS,
      THE CONTINUED USE MAY LEAD TO CUMULATIVE POISONING WHICH
      CAN BE COUNTERACTED WITH:
      A. Thrombin   D. Gamma globulin
      B. Protamine sulfate   E. Heparin
      C. Vitamin K

877. THE AVERAGE DIGITALIZING DOSE OF DIGOXIN IS:
      A. 1.0 gm.   D. 0.1 gm.
      B. 1.0 mg.   E. 1.0 grain
      C. 10.0 gm.

878. ALTERNATE DAY STEROID THERAPY IS MOST USEFUL IN TREATING:
      A. Ulcers
      B. Carcinoma of the lung
      C. Insulin shock
      D. Asthma
      E. Corneal ulcers

879.   ONE OF EPINEPHRINE'S ACTIONS ON THE HEART IS:
        A. Acceleration due to depression of the vagus
        B. Increase in refractory period
        C. Depression of the S.A. node
        D. Increase in the concentration of the enzyme phosphorylase A
        E. None of these

880.   EPINEPHRINE HCl HAS LITTLE OR NO EFFECT ON:
        A. Unbroken skin   D. Nasal mucosa
        B. Conjunctiva   E. Pupil
        C. Precapillary sphincter

881.   EPINEPHRINE HCl IS USED INTRAVENOUSLY IN CONCENTRATION OF:
        A. 1:100   D. 5%
        B. 1:1000   E. 10%
        C. 2%

882.   EPINEPHRINE IS OFTEN INCLUDED IN THE ADMINISTRATION OF LO-
        CAL ANESTHETICS BECAUSE IT:
        A. Enhances analgesic effect
        B. Neutralizes irritant action
        C. Delays diffusion of the anesthetic from the site of injection
        D. Increases diffusion of the anesthetic
        E. Increases blood levels of the anesthetic

883.   THE DISEASE MYRINGITIS INVOLVES THE:
        A. Stomach   D. Eye
        B. Intestines   E. Ear
        C. Nose

884.   RIFAMPIN MAY DO ALL OF THE FOLLOWING EXCEPT:
        A. Decrease BUN and serum uric acid
        B. Cause teratogenic effects
        C. Produce liver dysfunction
        D. Color urine and feces
        E. Inhibit effect of oral contraceptives

885.   WHICH TYPE OF PATIENT IS MOST LIKELY TO BE HYPERSENSITIVE
        TO ASPIRIN?
        A. Intrinsic asthmatic   D. Patient with viral infection
        B. Extrinsic asthmatic   E. C and D
        C. Chronic bronchitic

886.   THE PRINCIPAL ACTIVE ALKALOID OF IPECAC IS:
        A. Yohimbine   D. Lobeline
        B. Caffeine   E. Emetine
        C. Apomorphine

887.   EMETINE IS USED IN THE TREATMENT OF:
        A. Malaria
        B. Schistosomiasis
        C. Tuberculosis
        D. Amebiasis
        E. None of these

888. SENSITIZATION OF THE HEART TO EPINEPHRINE IS A POSSIBLE
DANGER IN THE USE OF:
A. Cyclopropane   D. Vinyl ether
B. Nitrous oxide   E. Pentothal
C. Ether

889. THE THERAPEUTIC USE OF NEOSTIGMINE BROMIDE IS AS:
A. Miotic   D. Neuromuscular blocker
B. CNS depressant   E. Muscle relaxant
C. Treatment for myasthenia gravis

890. ETHYLENEDIAMINETETRAACETIC ACID IS AN ANTIDOTE FOR
WHICH OF THE FOLLOWING?
A. Sodium secobarbital   D. Phosphorus
B. Aspirin   E. Lead
C. Paris green

891. THE DAILY MAINTENANCE DOSE OF CHLORAMPHENICOL IS
APPROXIMATELY:
A. 1.0 mg./kg. body weight
B. 5.0 mg./kg. body weight
C. 10.0 mg./kg. body weight
D. 20.0 mg./kg. body weight
E. 50.0 mg./kg. body weight

892. WHICH ONE OF THE FOLLOWING DRUGS REQUIRES REPEATED
PROTHROMBIN TIME DETERMINATIONS DURING ITS ADMINISTRATION?
A. Heparin   D. Protamine
B. Dicumarol   E. Regitine
C. Quinidine

893. THE ANTISPASMODIC ACTION OF PAPAVERINE ON SMOOTH MUSCLE
IS EXERTED:
A. Via stimulation of parasympathetic ganglia in intestinal wall
B. Via stimulation of sympathetic ganglia in intestinal wall
C. Directly on muscle cell
D. Through central nervous system
E. By parasympathetic blocking action

894. THE DRUG OF CHOICE IN TREATMENT OF VENTRICULAR TACHY-
CARDIA IS:
A. Quinidine   D. Methacholine (Mecholyl)
B. Digitoxin   E. Epinephrine
C. Digoxin

895. SIDE EFFECTS DUE TO ADMINISTRATION OF GANGLIONIC BLOCKING
DRUGS FOR THE TREATMENT OF HYPERTENSION DO NOT INCLUDE:
A. Constipation
B. Urinary retention
C. Impairment of visual accommodation
D. Profuse sweating
E. Dryness of mouth

896.   A SERIOUS CONSEQUENCE FROM CHRONIC USE OF THE "COAL TAR
        ANALGESICS" IS:
        A. Agranulocytosis   D. Aplastic anemia
        B. Leukemia   E. Carboxyhemoglobinemia
        C. Methemoglobinemia

897.   ISOETHARINE IS A DRUG WHICH STIMULATES PRIMARILY _____
        RECEPTORS.
        A. Alpha   D. Beta 2
        B. Histamine   E. None of the above
        C. Beta 1

898.   INCREASED CATECHOLAMINES IN THE URINE ARE DIAGNOSTIC OF:
        A. Cushing's syndrome   D. Amyloidosis
        B. Carcinoid syndrome   E. Pheochromocytoma
        C. Hyperparathyroidism

899.   THE PRIMARY USE OF METHOXYFLURANE IS AS A(N):
        A. Anesthetic   D. Hypnotic
        B. Analgesic   E. Hypotensive agent
        C. Cardiac stimulant

900.   IN CASE OF ACUTE PAIN OF ANGINA PECTORIS THE MOST EFFECTIVE
        TREATMENT WOULD BE TO ADMINISTER:
        A. Mannitol hexanitrate   D. Pentaerythritol tetranitrate
        B. Erythrityl tetranitrate   E. Nitroglycerin
        C. Sodium nitrite

901.   THE MECHANISM EXPLAINING THE CLINICAL PICTURE OBSERVED IN
        CARBON MONOXIDE POISONING IS:
        A. Hemolysis of red blood cells
        B. A chemical union of the carbon monoxide with the hemoglobin of the
            red blood cells
        C. Transformation of the carbon monoxide to carbon dioxide in the blood
        D. Arrest of oxidation in the tissues by enzyme interference
        E. None of the above

902.   CHLORAMPHENICOL IS PARTICULARLY EFFECTIVE IN THE TREAT-
        MENT OF:
        A. Diphtheria   D. Rickettsial diseases
        B. Tuberculosis   E. Strep. pyogenes infections
        C. Emphysema

903.   THE THERAPY OF CHOICE IN SCURVY IS:
        A. Vitamin D   D. Folic acid
        B. Vitamin B_2 E. Choline
        C. Vitamin C

904.   HEPARIN THERAPY IS BEST CONTROLLED WITH:
        A. Prothrombin time
        B. Platelet counts
        C. Bleeding times
        D. Clotting times
        E. No controls are needed

905. PILOCARPINE WOULD PRODUCE WHICH OF THE FOLLOWING?
A. Constriction of pupil of the eye   D. Tachycardia
B. Mydriasis   E. None of these
C. Cycloplegia

906. THE AVERAGE DAILY MAINTENANCE DOSE OF DIGITOXIN IS:
A. 0.1 gm.   D. 0.2 mg.
B. 0.2 gm.   E. 0.5 mg.
C. 0.1 mg.

907. THE DRUG OF CHOICE FOR SCARLET FEVER IS:
A. Tetracycline   D. Chloromycetin
B. Sulfonamides   E. Novobiocin
C. Penicillin

908. WHICH OF THE FOLLOWING IS THE MOST RAPID-ACTING DIGITALIS
PREPARATION?
A. Ouabain   D. Digitalis leaf
B. Digoxin   E. Lanatoside C
C. Digitoxin

909. ACETYLCHOLINE HAS BOTH MUSCARINIC AND NICOTINIC ACTIONS;
THE MUSCARINIC ACTION CAN BE BLOCKED BY:
A. Epinephrine   D. Curare
B. Atropine   E. Nicotine and curare
C. Nicotine

910. WHICH IS NOT AN ESTROGENIC SUBSTANCE?
A. Estradiol   D. Follicle stimulating hormone
B. Premarin   E. Stilbesterol
C. Theelin

911. SULFONAMIDES ARE EXCRETED FREE AND COMBINED AS THE:
A. Acetyl derivative   D. Glycine conjugate
B. Amino derivative   E. None of these
C. Sulfate derivative

912. TRIPLE SULFAS HAVE BEEN USED IN PREFERENCE TO SINGLE
SULFONAMIDES BECAUSE OF:
A. Synergistic action
B. Higher concentration in blood is obtained
C. They can be used in lower doses
D. Independent solubility of each sulfonamide
E. None of these

913. AN ANTIFUNGAL THAT RELEASES ACETIC ACID ONLY IN THE
PRESENCE OF FUNGUS IS:
A. Enzactin
B. Desenex
C. Vioform
D. Grisactin
E. Mycostatin

914. _____ IS THE FASTEST ACTING ANTICOAGULANT.
    A. Warfarin (Coumadin)   D. Protamine sulfate
    B. Heparin   E. Vitamin K
    C. Ouabain

915. AN ADVANTAGE OF EPHEDRINE SULFATE OVER EPINEPHRINE IS THAT:
    A. It is nontoxic
    B. It is more potent
    C. It is effective orally
    D. It decreases skeletal muscle tone
    E. It is more soluble

916. MEPERIDINE PRODUCES ANALGESIA EQUAL TO THAT OF MORPHINE IN A DOSE _____ THAT OF MORPHINE.
    A. 1/2   D. 100 times
    B. 8-10 times   E. 1/10
    C. Equal

917. WHICH OF THE FOLLOWING IS A GAMETOCIDAL AGENT IN MALARIA?
    A. Atabrine   D. Primaquine
    B. Quinine   E. Aralen
    C. Paludrine

918. WHICH OF THE FOLLOWING IS CONTRAINDICATED IN PATIENTS WITH HYPERTENSION AND EDEMA?
    A. Diazepoxide   D. Normal saline injection
    B. Furosemide   E. Chlorothiazide
    C. Hydrochlorothiazide

919. EXCESSIVE USE OF TOLBUTAMIDE WILL LEAD TO:
    A. Diarrhea   D. Acidosis
    B. Prolonged hypoglycemia   E. Glycosuria
    C. Tolerance to alcohol

920. WHICH OF THE FOLLOWING IS CONTRAINDICATED IN THE PRESENCE OF ACTIVE TUBERCULOSIS?
    A. Hydrocortisone   D. PAS
    B. Streptomycin   E. PABA
    C. INH

921. WHICH DOES DEMEROL NOT DEPRESS?
    A. Cough reflex   D. GI tract
    B. Ureter   E. Gall bladder
    C. Bladder

922. THE MAJOR DISADVANTAGE IN THE USE OF MEPERIDINE IS THAT IT PRODUCES:
    A. Low blood pressure
    B. High blood pressure
    C. Addiction
    D. Miosis
    E. Severe respiratory depression

923.   PARKINSONISM IS PROBABLY DUE TO:
     A. Too little dopamine in the brain
     B. Too little levodopa in the brain
     C. Too little acetylcholine in the brain
     D. Too much levodopa in the brain
     E. Too much dopamine in the brain

924.   A GROUP OF AGENTS USED PRIMARILY FOR BREAST
     CARCINOMAS ARE:
     A. Androgens   D. Digitalis glycosides
     B. Estrogens   E. Veratrum alkaloids
     C. Ethylaminobenzoates

925.   AN OVERDOSE OF d-TUBOCURARINE:
     A. Interferes with oxidative enzymes of the cells
     B. Paralyzes respiratory muscles
     C. May be combatted with carbachol
     D. Paralyzes the autonomic nervous system
     E. Depresses the medullary respiratory center

926.   ALL ANTIHISTAMINES APPEAR TO ANTAGONIZE HISTAMINE BY:
     A. Blocking release of histamine from mast cells
     B. Histaminase action
     C. Blocking synthesis of histamine
     D. Competing with histamine for cell receptors
     E. None of the above

927.   CODEINE ACTS AS A COUGH SEDATIVE BY:
     A. Producing mild nausea
     B. Depressing bronchiolar secretions
     C. Decreasing pulmonary action
     D. Depressing cough center
     E. Paralyzing sensory nerves of bronchi

928.   THE PHARMACOLOGICAL ACTION OF CASCARA SAGRADA IS
     LARGELY DUE TO:
     A. Hydrophilic action
     B. Capacity to swell and increase
     C. Antispasmodic action
     D. Mild irritating effect on intestine
     E. Central nervous system stimulation

929.   THE CHEMICAL PRECURSOR OF HISTAMINE IS:
     A. Hyaluronidase   D. Histidine
     B. Glycine   E. Epinephrine
     C. Glutamic acid

930.   PHENOTHIAZINES ARE NOT EFFECTIVE IN CONTROL OF
     VOMITING DUE TO:
     A. Radiation
     B. Infection
     C. Digitalis
     D. Upset stomach
     E. Motion sickness

931. THE GREATEST THREAT FROM MORPHINE POISONING IS:
    A. Renal shutdown   D. Cardiovascular collapse
    B. Paralysis of spinal cord   E. None of these
    C. Respiratory depression

932. ANTICOAGULANTS ARE USED IN THE TREATMENT OF:
    A. Peripheral vascular diseases   D. All of these
    B. Frostbite   E. None of these
    C. Prophylaxis of thrombophlebitis

933. WHICH OF THE FOLLOWING DOES NOT HAVE ANTIHISTAMINIC
    ACTION ?
    A. Neo-antergen   D. Diphenhydramine
    B. Chlorpromazine   E. Dilantin
    C. Pyribenzamine

934. AMMONIUM CHLORIDE IS USED TO INCREASE THE DIURETIC EFFECT
    OF WHICH OF THE FOLLOWING ?
    A. Xanthines   D. Diamox
    B. Urea   E. None of these
    C. Organic mercurials

935. THE DOSAGE RANGE AT WHICH AMPHETAMINE PRODUCES ITS
    THERAPEUTIC ACTION IS:
    A. 2.5-10 mg.   D. 25-50 mg.
    B. 0.05-0.25 mg.   E. 25-100 mg.
    C. 2.5-10 gm.

936. _____IS A SPECIFIC NARCOTIC ANTAGONIST.
    A. Meperidine   D. Universal antidote
    B. Polybrene   E. Meprobamate
    C. Nalorphine

937. WHICH OF THE FOLLOWING IS NOT A SIGN OF ACUTE MORPHINE
    POISONING ?
    A. Slow respiration   D. Hyperexia
    B. Pin-point pupils   E. Muscular flaccidity
    C. Oliguria

938. A VERY COMMON SIDE EFFECT OF MORPHINE IS:
    A. Allergic response   D. Liver damage
    B. Blood dyscrasias   E. Visceral pain
    C. Constipation

939. _____IS USED TO CURTAIL CHRONIC URIC ACID STONE
    FORMATION.
    A. Allopurinol
    B. Trimethoprim
    C. Methenamine
    D. Ethacrynic acid
    E. Furosemide

940. PUPILLARY CONSTRICTION BY MORPHINE IS:
  A. Due to local action on pupillary sphincter muscle
  B. No longer evident as tolerance develops
  C. Accompanied by increased intraocular pressure
  D. Overcome by atropine
  E. Due to action on medullary centers

941. A PROMINENT TOXIC EFFECT OF LOCAL ANESTHETICS IS:
  A. CNS stimulation
  B. CNS depression
  C. Tachycardia
  D. Local ischemia
  E. None of these

942. AMONG THE SIGNS OF BARBITURATE POISONING ARE:
  A. Hypertension
  B. Diuresis
  C. Decreased respiratory minute volume
  D. Alkalosis
  E. None of these

943. A DRUG WHICH COMBINES ANALGESIC ACTIVITY WITH MUSCLE RELAXANT PROPERTIES IS:
  A. Amobarbital
  B. Phenacetin
  C. Carisoprodol
  D. d-propoxyphene
  E. Aspirin

944. MONOAMINE OXIDASE PLAYS A ROLE IN THE METABOLISM OF:
  A. Serotonin
  B. Norepinephrine
  C. Acetylcholine
  D. A and B
  E. A and C

945. WHICH OF THE FOLLOWING IS CHARACTERISTIC OF VASOPRESSIN?
  A. Antidiuretic effect
  B. Constricts capillaries
  C. Coronary vasoconstriction
  D. Increased motility of bowel
  E. All of the above

REVIEW

946. A POTENT TRANQUILIZER WHICH ALSO EXHIBITS STRONG HYPOTENSIVE EFFECTS IS:
  A. Librium
  B. Meprobamate
  C. Reserpine
  D. Thorazine
  E. Sparine

947. _____ IS USED TO LOWER BLOOD LIPID LEVELS.
  A. Trimethadione
  B. Clofibrate
  C. Flucytosine
  D. Coumarin
  E. Propranolol

948. FURADANTIN IS USED MAINLY FOR:
  A. Amebic dysentery
  B. Genito-urinary infections
  C. Resistant staph infections
  D. Pneumococcal infections
  E. None of the above

78

SECTION II - PHARMACOLOGY

CHECK OUT MATCH THE FOLLOWING:

949. D   Reserpine
950. C   Meprobamate
951. A   Iproniazid
952. E   Chlorpromazine
953. B   Mescaline

A. Inhibits monoamine oxidase
B. Hallucinogenic drug
C. Convulsions may occur in withdrawal
D. Releases norepinephrine from brain
E. Parkinsonism occurs with high doses

MATCH THE FOLLOWING:

954. E   Scopolamine
955. D   Homatropine
956. B   Amphetamine
957. C   Prednisone
958. A   Isoproterenol

A. To reverse acute asthmatic attack
B. To control appetite
C. To give prolonged suppression of
   angioneurotic edema
D. To produce mydriasis
E. To effect preanesthetic sedation

MATCH THE FOLLOWING:

959. E   Neomycin
960. C   Chloramphenicol
961. B   Tetracycline
962. D   Bacitracin
963. A   Nystatin

A. Effective in treatment of moniliasis
B. May be given I. M. or I. V. in severe
   acute infections
C. May cause aplastic anemia
D. Nephrotoxic
E. May cause permanent deafness if given
   parenterally

MATCH EACH DRUG WITH ITS PREVALENT ADVERSE EFFECT:

964. B   Indocin
965. E   Soma
966. D   Tetracycline
967. A   Sinutabs
968. C   Streptomycin

A. Light-headedness
B. Severe gastric upset
C. Tinnitis
D. Discoloration of teeth
E. Skin eruptions

969. WHICH OF THE FOLLOWING COULD BE USED AS AN ANTIDOTE
     FOR CURARE POISONING?
     A. Neostigmine
     B. Atropine
     C. Homatropine
     D. Hexamethonium
     E. None of the above

MATCH THE FOLLOWING:

970. B Quinine
971. D Quinacrine
972. E Primaquine
973. C Chloroquine
974. A Pamaquine

A. A highly toxic 8-aminoquinoline
B. Has action on striated muscle
C. Useful only against erythrocytic phase
   of disease
D. Acridine dye, which causes yellowing
   of skin
E. Effective in radical cure of vivax
   malaria

MATCH THE FOLLOWING:

975. B Trichloroethylene
976. C Nitrous oxide
977. D Cyclopropane
978. E Ethylene
979. A Divinyl ether

A. Useful for induction in patients with
   broncho-constriction
B. Tachypnea is a sign of overdosage
C. Will not produce adequate muscular
   relaxation
D. Gas with 100% potency
E. Relatively impotent and explosive

MATCH THE FOLLOWING:

980. C Barbital
981. B Phenobarbital
982. D Amobarbital
983. E Secobarbital
984. A Thiopental

A. Highly soluble in body fat
B. Produces specific corticomotor
   depression
C. No appreciable hepatic destruction
D. Intermediate duration of action
E. Not likely to produce a hangover

MATCH THE FOLLOWING:

985. C Atropine
986. A Epinephrine
987. D Carbachol
988. E Physostigmine
989. C Phenylephrine

A. Glycogenolysis
B. Increase in mean blood pressure with
   bradycardia
C. Mydriasis and anhydrosis
D. Cycloplegia without mydriasis
E. Used in treatment of paralytic ileus

990. THERAPEUTICALLY VITAMIN B1 HAS BEEN EMPLOYED MOST
      SUCCESSFULLY IN THE TREATMENT OF:
      A. Microcytic anemia   D. Beriberi
      B. Pellagra   E. Macrocytic anemia
      C. Scurvy

991. AMINOPHYLLINE IS USED MOST FREQUENTLY IN:
      A. Asthma
      B. Nephritic edema
      C. Lowering cerebral pressure
      D. Eliminating toxins in the body
      E. Diabetes insipidus

8
22

992.   PROPYLTHIOURACIL IS USEFUL IN THE TREATMENT OF:
       A.   Derangement toxicosis   D.   Hyperthyroidism
       B.   Hypothyroidism   E.   Thyroiditis
       C.   Hypoparathyroidism

993.   A SERIOUS SIDE EFFECT OF ALKERAN IS:
       A.   Phagocytosis
       B.   Tolerance develops rapidly
       C.   Depression of WBC
       D.   Severe kidney damage
       E.   Visual disturbances

MATCH THE FOLLOWING DRUGS WITH THE MOST CLOSELY RELATED
STATEMENT:

994.   C   Ergonovine   A.   An anticoagulant which interferes with
995.   D   Pamaquine   prothrombin synthesis
996.   E   6-Mercaptopurine   B.   A potent antihistamine
997.   A   Bishydroxycoumarin   C.   Used to control post partum bleeding
998.   B   Tripelennamine   D.   An antimalarial with gametocidal action
                                    E.   A nucleic acid anti-metabolite

MATCH THE FOLLOWING:

999.   B   Physostigmine   A.   Antihistamine drug
1000. A   Diphenhydramine   B.   Cholinesterase inhibitor
1001. C   Atropine   C.   Cholinergic blocking agent
1002. E   Nicotine   D.   Adrenergic blocking agent
1003. D   Ergotamine   E.   Ganglionic stimulating agent

1004. YELLOW PIGMENTATION OF THE SKIN IS MOST COMMON WITH:
       A.   Chloraquine
       B.   Pamaquin
       C.   Quinicrine
       D.   Quinine
       E.   Atabrine

MATCH THE FOLLOWING:

1005. D   Codeine   A.   Used in treatment of addiction
1006. E   Papaverine   B.   Analgesic with some antispasmodic action
1007. B   Meperidine   C.   Most abundant alkaloid in opium
1008. A   Methadone   D.   Weakest of the phenanthrene analgesics
1009. C   Morphine   E.   No antagonism by nalorphine

1010. ALL BUT ONE ARE SPASTIC DISEASES OF THE BLOOD VESSELS:
       A.   Angina pectoris
       B.   Migraine
       C.   Ergot poisoning
       D.   Raynaud's disease
       E.   Tetanus

13
/ 9

MATCH THE FOLLOWING:

1011. _D_ Magnesium trisilicate   A. Increases myocardial force
1012. _C_ Magnesium sulfate   B. Central nervous system stimulant
1013. _B_ Metrazol   C. Saline cathartic
1014. _E_ Nalline HCL   D. Gastric antacid, absorbent
1015. _A_ Digitoxin   E. Narcotic antagonist

1016. NOREPINEPHRINE IN THERAPEUTIC DOSAGE RAISES THE BLOOD
PRESSURE IN ASSOCIATION WITH:
A. Unchanged peripheral vascular resistance and tachycardia
B. Reduced peripheral vascular resistance and unchanged pulse rate
C. Increased peripheral vascular resistance and tachycardia
D. Increased peripheral vascular resistance and bradycardia
E. None of the above

1017. SPIRONOLACTONE ACTS BY ANTAGONIZING:
A. Insulin
B. Glucagon
C. Aldosterone
D. Histamine
E. A and C

1018. WHICH ONE OF THE FOLLOWING DOES NOT REPRESENT AN ACTION
OF QUINIDINE ON THE MYOCARDIUM?
A. Increases the refractory period
B. Increases force of contraction of the muscle
C. Raises the fibrillation threshold
D. Blocks vagal effects on heart
E. Slows conduction

1019. WHICH OF THE FOLLOWING DOES NOT ENHANCE THE POTENTIAL
TOXIC EFFECTS OF DIGITALIS ON THE HEART?
A. Increased renal clearance   D. Low serum potassium
B. Myocardial anoxia   E. High serum calcium
C. Alkalosis

1020. THE BETA-ADRENERGIC RECEPTOR IS:
A. Activated most prominently by norepinephrine
B. Blocked by adrenergic blocking agents
C. Found only in cardiac muscle
D. Associated primarily with inhibitory responses
E. Not stimulated by isopropylarterenol

1021. THE EFFECTS OF PROPYLTHIOURACIL MEDICATION MAY NOT
APPEAR FOR SEVERAL DAYS BECAUSE:
A. The dose is small
B. The drug is only partially absorbed
C. 70% of the drug is inactivated by the gastric juices
D. Stored thyroxin is present in the gland
E. Its action is cumulative

1022. WHICH IS NOT A NOTICEABLE EFFECT OF DIGITOXIN IN CARDIAC
       FAILURE?
       A. Increased venous pressure
       B. Increased urinary output
       C. Retarded A-V conduction
       D. Decreased diastolic size of heart
       E. Increased cardiac output

       MATCH THE FOLLOWING:

1023. E Ergonovine   A. Sedative, hypnotic, mydriatic
1024. C Heparin sodium   B. Antibiotic effecting gram positive
1025. A Hyoscine hydrobromide   bacteria
1026. B Erythromycin   C. Increases blood coagulation time
1027. D Methyltestosterone   D. Male hormone
                                  E. Oxytocic

1028. WHICH IS THE DRUG OF CHOICE FOR TRIGEMINAL NEURALGIA?
       A. Carbamazepine
       B. Phenytoin
       C. Flurazepam
       D. Diazepam
       E. Trimethadione

1029. THE MOST EFFECTIVE DRUG FOR PROPHYLAXIS AGAINST
       MENINGITIS IS:
       A. Penicillin G
       B. Penicillin V
       C. Tetracycline
       D. Erythromycin
       E. Sulfisoxazole

1030. _____C_____ MAY INCREASE SEIZURE ACTIVITY IN EPILEPTIC PATIENTS.
       A. Ethotoin   D. Amantadine
       B. Phenobarbital   E. L-Dopa
       C. Trihexyphenidyl

1031. THE THERAPEUTIC USE OF NEOSTIGMINE BROMIDE IS AS:
       A. Miotic   D. Diaphoretic
       B. Nerve sedative   E. Vasoconstrictor
       C. Therapy of myasthenia gravis

1032. _____ IS SOMETIMES USED TO PROMOTE CONVULSIONS
       IN EXPERIMENTAL ANIMALS.
       A. Dilantin
       B. Mephenesin
       C. Phenobarbital
       D. Strychnine
       E. Methadone

1033.   PHARMACOLOGICAL EFFECTS OF HEXAMETHONIUM ARE CENTERED
        CHIEFLY ON:
        A. Autonomic ganglia
        B. Parasympathetic nerve endings
        C. Adrenal medulla
        D. Sympathetic nerve endings
        E. Neuromuscular junction

1034.   HYCODAN (HYDROCODONE BITARTRATE) ACTS AS A COUGH SEDATIVE
        BY:
        A. Producing mild nausea
        B. Depressing bronchiolar secretions
        C. Diminishing bronchiolar secretions
        D. Depressing cough center
        E. Paralyzing sensory nerve of bronchi

1035.   METHYSERGIDE IS USED PRIMARILY TO TREAT:
        A. Grand mal epilepsy
        B. Petit mal epilepsy
        C. Focal epilepsy
        D. Migraine headache
        E. Hypertension

        MATCH THE FOLLOWING:

1036. C Thiopental   A. Synthetic analgesic useful in labor
1037. A Meperidine   B. Produces a hypotensive action by
1038. D Ephedrine   peripheral vasodilation
1039. E Hexamethonium   C. Rapid-acting barbiturate
1040. B Hydralazine   D. Long-acting sympathomimetic drug
                               E. Ganglionic blocking agent for use in
                                   hypertension

1041.   THE PRINICIPAL DIFFERENCE BETWEEN COMPETITIVE AND NON-
        COMPETITIVE INHIBITION IS:
        A. Extent of receptor site blockage   D. Degree of agonism
        B. Whether inhibition occurs   E. None of the above
        C. Extent of enzyme inhibition

1042.   WHICH IS NOT A CONTRAINDICATION FOR BARBITURATES?
        A. Insomnia   D. Drug addiction
        B. Severe kidney disease   E. Alcoholism
        C. Diabetes

1043.   THE MERCURIAL DIURETICS INCREASE THE FLOW OF URINE BY:
        A. Increasing filtration pressure
        B. Increasing capillary permeability
        C. Increasing selective resorption
        D. Increasing resorption through Henle's loop
        E. None of these

1044.   A CLASS OF PLANT ALKALOIDS THAT ARE WIDELY USED TO TREAT
         MIGRAINE ARE:
         A. Vinca alkaloids
         B. Digitalis glycosides
         C. Stramonium alkaloids
         D. Ergot alkaloids
         E. Belladonna alkaloids

         MATCH THE FOLLOWING:

1045. _D_ Preludin   A. Coronary vasodilator
1046. _A_ Nitroglycerin   B. Antihypertensive
1047. _E_ Levophed   C. General anesthetic
1048. _B_ Ismelin   D. Appetite suppressant
1049. _C_ Cyclopropane   E. To treat shock

1050.   ALCOHOL HALLUCINOSIS IS COMMONLY TREATED WITH:
         A. Disulfiram (Antabuse)
         B. Phenothiazines
         C. Barbiturates
         D. Caffeine
         E. Oxygen

         MATCH EACH DRUG WITH ITS USUAL DOSE:

1051. _C_ Emetine (IM)   A. 150 mg.
1052. _A_ Declomycin   B. 1-4 mg.
1053. _B_ Stelazine   C. 1 mg./Kg.
1054. _E_ Povan   D. 100 mg.
1055. _D_ Nembutal   E. 5 mg./Kg.

1056.   A TOXIC EFFECT OF ALCOHOL IS:
         A. Mitosis   D. CNS stimulation
         B. Mydriasis   E. Respiratory depression
         C. Agranulocytosis

1057.   WHICH OF THE FOLLOWING IS A SEROTONIN ANTAGONIST ?
         A. Glutethimide   D. Tripelennamine
         B. Caffeine   E. Methysergide
         C. Tolbutamide

1058.   BISACODYL FREQUENTLY CAN CAUSE:
         A. Abdominal cramps
         B. Constipation
         C. Skin rashes
         D. Dizziness
         E. Nausea

FOUR CONDITIONS ARE LISTED BELOW IN COLUMN II. ASSOCIATE
EACH WITH ONE OF THE DRUGS LISTED IN COLUMN I:

COLUMN I   COLUMN II

1059. B Acetylsalicylic acid   A. Agranulocytosis
1060. D Acetanilid   B. Respiratory alkalosis
1061. A Aminopyrine   C. Toxic cirrhosis of the liver
                                      D. Methemoglobinemia

MATCH THE FOLLOWING CONDITIONS WITH THE DRUG OF
CHOICE:

1062. D Narcotic overdosage   A. Indomethacin
1063. C Pinworms   B. Chloramphenicol
1064. B Typhoid fever   C. Pyrvinium pamoate
1065. A Arthritis   D. Nalorphine

RELATE THE FOLLOWING:

1066. E Triiodothyronine   A. Causes involution of thyroid gland with
1067. D Thyrotropic hormone   colloid storage
1068. C Thiouracil   B. Does not prevent iodide uptake
1069. A Iodide   C. Suppresses thyroxin formation and
                                   decreases amount of colloid in thyroid
                                   gland
                                D. Stimulates release and synthesis of
                                   thyroxin
                                E. More potent than thyroxin

RELATE THE FOLLOWING:

1070. A Action of mecholyl on cardiac   A. Rate of diastolic depolari-
         pacemaker   zation decreased
1071. C Action of procaine on nerve   B. Miniature e.p.p. reduced
1072. B Action of tubocurarine at motor C. Membrane potential
         end plate   stabilized

RELATE THE FOLLOWING:

A. Cocaine
B. Curare
C. Botulinus toxin
D. Eserine

1073. D Potentiates response of intestinal muscle to acetylcholine
1074. A Potentiates the response of smooth muscle to epinephrine
1075. C Blocks liberation of acetylcholine at nerve endings
1076. B Decreases amplitude and frequency of spontaneous "miniature" end
         plate potentials

LOOK UP

RELATE THE FOLLOWING:

1077.	C Tribromoethanol	A.	Used in trigeminal neuralgia
1078.	E Chloroform	B.	Produces local anesthesia by freezing
1079.	F Ether	C.	Basal anesthetic
1080.	B Ethyl chloride	D.	Very rapid induction
1081.	A Trichlorethylene	E.	Sensitizes heart to epinephrine
1082.	D Vinyl ether	F.	Has curariform action
1083.	I Nitrous oxide	G.	Most potent gaseous anesthetic
1084.	H Ethylene	H.	Almost no cardiovascular action
1085.	G Cyclopropane	I.	Greatest danger associated with its use is anoxia

MATCH THE STATEMENT WITH THE MOST APPROPRIATE DRUG
USING EACH ANSWER ONLY ONCE:

1086.	B Inhibited by PABA	A.	Polymyxin
1087.	C Skin eruptions are the most common type of allergic response	B.	Sulfonamides
1088.	D Eradicates both cysts and trophozoites of intestinal amebiasis from the feces	C.	Penicillin
		D.	Tetracycline
1089.	A Neurotoxic upon parenteral administration	E.	Sulfones
1090.	F Equal or superior to streptomycin as an anti-tubercular drug	F.	Isoniazid
1091.	E Drug of choice for Hansen's disease		

LOOK UP

RELATE THE FOLLOWING:

1092.	B Urethane	A.	Toxic effects overcome by citrovorum factor
1093.	A Aminopterin		
1094.	E Myleran	B.	Drug of choice in multiple myeloma
1095.	D 6-Mercaptopurine	C.	Should only be given I. V.
1096.	C Mechlorethamine	D.	May be incorporated into RNA and DNA
		E.	Cytotoxic action largely limited to bone marrow

MATCH THE FOLLOWING DISEASE OR CONDITION WITH THE DRUG
USED TO TREAT IT:

1097.	C Diabetes	A.	Allopurinol
1098.	D Hay Fever	B.	Chlorpromazine
1099.	B Nausea	C.	Tolbutamide
1100.	F Migraine	D.	Diphenhydramine
1101.	E Epilepsy	E.	Diphenylhydantoin
1102.	A Gout	F.	Ergotamine
1103.	G Insomnia	G.	Pentobarbital
1104.	H Obesity	H.	Amphetamines

12
20

MATCH EACH DRUG WITH THE APPROPRIATE USE:

1105. C Pancuronium (Pavulon)   A. Anesthetic
1106. D Pentazocine (Talwin)   B. Narcotic antagonist
1107. A Ketamine   C. Muscle relaxation
1108. B Naloxone (Narcan)   D. Analgesic
1109. F Amantadine (Symmetrel)   E. Anticoagulant
1110. E Phenindione (Hedulin)   F. Anti-viral
1111. G Propranolol (Inderal)   G. Anti-arrhythmic

CHOOSE THE NEAREST CORRECT AVERAGE ADULT ORAL DOSES
FOR THE FOLLOWING DRUGS (SOME ANSWERS MAY BE USED MORE
THAN ONCE):

1112. D Acetylsalicylic acid (analgesic)   A. 0.5 mg.
1113. F Phenobarbital   B. 1.0 gm.
1114. A Reserpine   C. 0.5 gm.
1115. E Atropine   D. 0.3 gm.
1116. A Glyceryl trinitrate   E. 0.02 mg.
1117. B Procainamide (for ventricular   F. 15 mg.
          tachycardia)   G. 15 gm.
1118. C Chlorothiazide
1119. F Ethinylestradiol (in menopause)
1120. G Magnesium sulfate (cathartic)

1121.   A COMMON SIDE EFFECT ON EPHEDRINE IS:
         A. Rashes   D. Drowsiness
         B. Nervousness   E. Ulcers
         C. Blood Dyscrasias

1122.   A SERIOUS SIDE EFFECT OF PHENOTHIAZINE DERIVATIVES IS:
         A. Increase heart rate markedly   D. Shock
         B. Agranulocytosis   E. Brain damage
         C. Respiratory interference

WHICH STATEMENT IN COLUMN II BEST DESCRIBES THE DRUG
IN COLUMN I:

COLUMN I   COLUMN II

1123. A Meprobamate   A. A propanediol derivative related to
1124. D Azacyclonal   mephenesin
1125. E Methylphenidate   B. Antagonizes psychologic effect of LSD
1126. D Reserpine   in humans
1127. C Chlorpromazine   C. A phenothiazine compound with
                                    "tranquilizing" action
                                D. A tranquilizer with an indole moiety
                                    in its structure
                                E. A piperidine derivative which elevates
                                    mood of depressed patients

18
23

RELATE THE FOLLOWING DRUGS TO THE CORRECT ROUTE OF
METABOLISM OR METABOLIC PRODUCT:

1128. C	Salicylates	A.	Side chain oxidation in liver
1129. E	Epinephrine	B.	Trichlorethanol glucuronide
1130. J	Ether	C.	Gentisic acid
1131. A	Phenobarbital	D.	Methyluric acid
1132. F	Serotonin	E.	Methylation of orthohydroxy group
1133. G	Succinylcholine	F.	5-OH indoleacetic acid
1134. H	Sulfonamides	G.	Hydrolysis by plasma cholinesterase
1135. B	Chloral hydrate	H.	Acetylation
1136. D	Caffeine	I.	Sulfoxide formation
1137. I	Chlorpromazine	J.	Excreted via lungs unchanged

A SKELETAL MUSCLE IS STIMULATED THROUGH ITS NERVE AT A
RATE OF ONE MAXIMAL SHOCK PER FIVE SECONDS. PARTIAL
PARALYSIS IS THEN PRODUCED WITH ONE OF THE DRUGS LISTED
BELOW. A TETANIC STIMULUS IS THEN APPLIED AT A RATE OF
50 SHOCKS PER SECOND FOR 2 SECONDS. AFTER THE TETANIC
STIMULATION SINGLE SHOCKS ARE RESUMED. THREE TYPES OF
RESPONSE ARE OBSERVED DEPENDING UPON THE TYPE OF DRUG
USED. MATCH THE CORRECT RESPONSE WITH THE DRUGS LISTED:

A 1138. C   Tetraethylpyrophosphate   A. Paralysis intensified
B 1139. C   Benzoquinonium   B. Paralysis diminished
B 1140. C   Gallamine   C. No effect
A 1141. C   Edrophonium (large dose)
  1142. B   Curare
A 1143. C   Octamethyl pyrophosphoramide
A 1144. C   Decamethonium (early phase of block)
C 1145. B   Botulinus toxin
A 1146. C   Succinylcholine (early phase of block)
A 1147. A   DFP

MATCH THE STATEMENT WITH THE MOST APPROPRIATE DRUG
USING EACH ANSWER ONLY ONCE:

A. Phenacemid (Phenurone)
B. Diphenylhydantoin (Dilantin)
C. Pentylenetetrazol (Metrazol)
D. Methylphenylethylhydantoin (Mesantoin)
E. Paramethadione (Paradione)
F. Primidone (Mysoline)

1148. B   Effective against grand mal seizures
1149. F   Effective against petit mal seizures
1150. E   One of the most toxic of the clinically available antiepileptics
1151. A   Intensifies the preictal aura
1152. D   Combined use with trimethadione or paramethadione is especially
          prone to cause severe toxic reactions
1153. C   A central nervous system stimulant

KNOW

RELATE THE FOLLOWING:

- 1154. E   EDTA
- 1155. G   Aminopterin
- 1156. B   BAL
- 1157. D   Bretylium
- 1158. H   Sodium nitrite
- 1159. A   Dibenamine
- 1160. J   Tetraethylthiuram disulfide
- 1161. C   Oxytocin
- 1162. F   Diamox (acetazolamide)
- 1163. I   Atropine

A. Antagonist to norepinephrine
B. Antidote of mercuhydrin
C. Direct action on uterine musculature
D. Inhibits release of norepinephrine
   from adrenergic nerves
E. Given I.V. as Ca, Na salt
F. Carbonic anhydrase inhibitor
G. Folic acid antagonist
H. Antidote for cyanide
I. DFP antidote
J. Inhibits oxidation of alcohol

MATCH EACH DRUG WITH ITS PREVALENT SIDE EFFECT:

1164. C   Reserpine
1165. B   Mercurophylline
1166. A   Morphine
1167. E   Thioridazine
1168. F   Dimenhydrinate

A. Constipation
B. Respiratory distress
C. Postural hypotension
D. Stomatitis
E. Agranulocytosis
F. Drowsiness

MATCH THE FOLLOWING DRUGS WITH THEIR PRIMARY
PHARMACOLOGICAL ACTION:

1169. C   Colchicine
1170. E   Digitalis
1171. A   Griseofulvin
1172. B   Tripelennamine
1173. D   Ethchlorvynol

A. Fungistatic activity
B. Antihistaminic activity
C. Uricosuric activity
D. Sedative activity
E. Cardiotonic activity

MATCH EACH DRUG WITH ITS USUAL AVERAGE ADULT DOSE:

1174. B   Dextropropoxyphene
1175. C   Declomycin
1176. A   Reserpine
1177. E   Pentobarbital
1178. D   Gantrisin

A. 0.25 mg.
B. 65 mg.
C. 150 mg.
D. 0.5 Gm.
E. 100 mg.

RELATE THE FOLLOWING:

1179. A   Amphetamine
1180. C   Carbamylcholine
1181. QB   Tolazoline
1182. D   Reserpine
1183. E   5-hydroxytryptamine

A. Sympathomimetic
B. Adrenergic blocking agent
C. Parasympathomimetic
D. Decreases catecholamine
   stored in tissues
E. None of these

19
—
50

1184. A MUSCLE RELAXANT WHOSE EFFECTS ARE LIMITED TO THE
       SPINAL CORD IS_____.
       A. Robaxin
       B. Rela
       C. Artane
       D. Pro-Banthine
       E. Sinaxar

1185. AN ADVANTAGE OF NORTRIPTYLINE (AVENTYL) OVER OTHER
       DIBENZAZEPINES IS IT _____.
       A. Has a longer duration of action A
       B. Is far less toxic
       C. Is more soluble
       D. Acts faster
       E. Is usually given parenterally

1186. THE MOST EFFECTIVE SINGLE CHEMOTHERAPEUTIC AGENT OF
       THOSE INDICATED, IN THE TREATMENT OF TUBERCULOSIS, IS:
       A. Neomycin   D. Penicillin
       B. Sulfones   E. Terramycin
       C. Streptomycin

1187. EUTONYL (PARGYLINE) IS SPECIFICALLY CONTRAINDICATED IN:
       A. Diabetes   D. Hyperthyroidism
       B. Hypertension   E. Heart disease
       C. Frostbite

1188. WHICH OF THE FOLLOWING STATEMENTS IS TRUE OF HEPARIN?
       A. Obtained from spoiled sweet clover
       B. Destroyed in intestinal tract
       C. Does not prevent clotting of shed blood
       D. Inhibits prothrombin synthesis in liver
       E. None of these

1189. WHICH OF THE FOLLOWING STATEMENTS IS TRUE OF BISHYDROXY-
       COUMARIN?
       A. Obtained from cattle lung
       B. Has antithrombin action
       C. Prevents clotting of shed blood
       D. Not antagonized by fresh whole blood
       E. None of these

1190. A DRUG USED IN TESTING FOR MYASTHENIA GRAVIS IS:
       A. Regitine
       B. Atropine
       C. Curare
       D. Edrophonium chloride (Tensilon)
       E. Decamethonium

1191. THE CHIEF USE OF LEVOARTERENOL IS TO TREAT_____.
       A. Shock
       B. Diabetes
       C. Hypertension
       D. Cardiac arrhythmias
       E. Iron deficiencies

1192.   TOLERANCE TO NITROGLYCERIN MAY BE OVERCOME BY:
         A. Initially using the largest safe dose of the drug
         B. Using other nitrites
         C. Temporarily discontinuing the drug for one or two weeks
         D. Use of higher doses
         E. None of the above

1193.   THE FIRST SYMPTOMS OF ACUTE POISONING WITH
         METHANOL ARE:
         A. G.I. and abdominal distress
         B. Delirium and restlessness
         C. Blurring or dimness of vision
         D. Oculogyric crises
         E. Muscle cramps and weakness

1194.   ETHACRYNIC ACID IS USED PRIMARILY AS A(AN):
         A. Diuretic
         B. Anti-emetic
         C. Laxative
         D. Sedative
         E. Analgesic

1195.   ANTIHISTAMINES HAVE LITTLE EFFECT ON WHICH ONE OF THE
         FOLLOWING ACTIONS OF HISTAMINE?
         A. Bronchospasm
         B. Wheal and flare
         C. Hypotension
         D. Gastric secretion
         E. Increased capillary permeability

1196.   ACUTE BRONCHIAL ASTHMA IS AN INDICATION FOR ALL BUT ONE
         OF THE FOLLOWING:
         A. Epinephrine
         B. Ephedrine
         C. Aminophylline
         D. Prednisolone
         E. Bradykinin

1197.   PARNATE EXERTS ITS ACTION BY:
         A. Producing epinephrine
         B. Inhibiting acetylcholine
         C. Inhibiting MAO
         D. Direct action on medulla
         E. Direct action on spinal cord

FOR THE FOLLOWING, LIST THE LETTER OF THE STATEMENT
WHICH IS TRUE WHEN APPLIED TO THE PARTICULAR DRUG LISTED:

1198.   AN ADVANTAGE OF DOPRAM OVER OTHER ANALEPTICS IS _____.
        A. Short duration of action
        B. Long duration of action
        C. It does not depress respiration
        D. Dosage easier to adjust
        E. None of the above

1199.   WHICH OF THE FOLLOWING IS USED TO RELIEVE GI MUSCLE SPASM?
        A. Edrophonium (Tensilon)
        B. Bethanechol (Urecholine)
        C. Guanethidine (Ismelin)
        D. Epinephrine
        E. Dicyclomine (Bentyl)

1200.   CHOOSE THE AGENT USED TO PREVENT LOCAL NECROSIS FROM
        NOREPINEPHRINE INFUSIONS:
        A. Propranolol (Inderal)
        B. Phentolamine (Regitine)
        C. Ephedrine
        D. Dopamine
        E. Edrophonium (Tensilon)

1201.   ISOXSUPRINE IS USED TO TREAT:
        A. Asthma
        B. Severe hypotension
        C. Nasal congestion
        D. Premature labor
        E. Hypertension

1202.   WHICH IS AN ANTIDOTE FOR MALATHION POISONING?
        A. Vitamin K
        B. Protamine sulfate
        C. Nalorphine (Nalline)
        D. Pralidoxime (Protopam)
        E. Edrophonium (Tensilon)

1203.   THE USUAL DOSAGE SCHEDULE OF THIAZIDE DIURETICS IS:
        A. Q. 4 h.
        B. Q. i. d.
        C. T. i. d.
        D. Weekly
        E. Once daily

1204.   A GROUP OF DRUGS USED WIDELY TO TREAT MILD HYPERTENSION
        IS:
        A. Sympathetic blockers
        B. Diuretics
        C. Ganglionic blockers
        D. MAO inhibitors
        E. None of the above

1205. METHYLPHENIDATE (RITALIN) DOES NOT:
A. Increase spontaneous activity in animals
B. Produce uncoordinated movements in normal dose range
C. Antagonize barbiturate depression
D. Affect mood of normal subjects
E. Elevate mood without producing euphoria

1206. A PROBLEM WHICH IS OFTEN SEEN WHEN MERCURIAL DIURETICS ARE GIVEN IS:
A. Anuria
B. Dizziness
C. Severe nausea
D. Acidosis
E. Alkalosis

1207. CODEINE DIFFERS CHEMICALLY FROM MORPHINE BY VIRTUE OF:
A. Methyl substitution on the alcoholic hydroxy group
B. Methyl substitution on both alcoholic and phenolic hydroxy group
C. Replacement of phenolic hydroxy group with an ethoxy group
D. Methylation of position 7 of the phenanthrene nucleus
E. None of these

1208. ETHACRYNIC ACID IS USED PRIMARILY AS A(N):
A. Cardiac glycoside
B. Agent to treat anorexia
C. Agent to treat hemophilia
D. Agent to treat gout
E. Diuretic

1209. WHAT IS THE CHIEF CONTRAINDICATION OF PARALDEHYDE?
A. Ulcers
B. Diabetics
C. Hepatic disease
D. Pregnant women
E. Ulcerative colitis

1210. THE EMERGENCY INTRAVENOUS DIGITALIZING DOSE OF OUABAIN IS APPROXIMATELY:
A. 0.25 to 0.5 mg.
B. 1.0 mg.
C. 5-10 mg.
D. 0.1 gm.
E. .01 mg.

MATCH THE FOLLOWING:

1211. ___ Purified protein derivative   A. Prepared in a special protein free
          of tuberculin   media
1212. ___ Rhus extracts   B. Prepared from human tubercle
1213. ___ Snake venom   bacillus
1214. ___ Old tuberculin   C. For immunization to poison ivy
1215. ___ B. C. G.   D. Used as an analgesic in intractable
                                            cancer pain
                                         E. Attenuated bovine tubercle bacilli

1216. ALUM PRECIPITATED DIPHTHERIA TOXOID:
       A. Retains toxicity in guinea pigs
       B. Contains about 20% of the protein in the original toxoid
       C. Contains serum albumin
       D. Is liberated slowly from the precipitate when injected
       E. Does not require booster shots

1217. SCARLET FEVER STREPTOCOCCUS TOXIN:
       A. Is used in Schick test
       B. Contains 10% peptone
       C. Contains a soluble toxin from the growth in broth of hemolytic
          streptococci
       D. May contain horse blood in the culture medium
       E. Causes Dick test to become positive when used prophylactically

1218. DIAGNOSTIC DIPHTHERIA TOXIN:
       A. Is used in Schick test
       B. Contains phenol as a bacteriostatic agent
       C. Is injected intradermally in an amount equivalent to 1 M. L. D. dose
          in a guinea pig
       D. Is injected intramuscularly
       E. Dose is 1. 0 cc.

1219. WHICH STATEMENT IS NOT TRUE OF TYPHOID AND PARATYPHOID
       VACCINE?
       A. Contains killed eberthella typhosa
       B. Contains killed Salmonella paratyphi
       C. Contains killed Salmonella schottmülleri
       D. Is known as triple vaccine
       E. Is prepared from a common culture of typhoid and paratyphoid
          organisms

1220. CHOLERA VACCINE:
       A. Contains at least 8000 million cholera organisms
       B. Is prepared from attenuated or killed vibrio comma
       C. Is a sterile suspension in isotonic sodium chloride
       D. All of these
       E. None of these

1221.   YELLOW FEVER VACCINE:
A.   Is a suspension in water for injection
B.   Consists of killed strain of yellow fever virus
C.   Is a living culture of an attenuated strain of yellow fever virus
D.   Requires no special labelling
E.   Imparts immunity which lasts for less than 1 year

1222.   EPIDEMIC TYPHUS VACCINE:
A.   Is obtained from rickettsia cultured from yolk sac membrane of developing embryo of domestic fowl
B.   Contains living attenuated rickettsia
C.   Does not require booster shots
D.   Provides only passive immunity
E.   None of these

MATCH THE FOLLOWING:

1223. ___   Bacteriolysins
1224. ___   Bacteriotropins
1225. ___   Opsonins
1226. ___   Agglutinins
1227. ___   Precipitins

A.   Precipitate solutions of bacterial substances
B.   Does not require complement
C.   Requires complement for bactericidal action
D.   Are not bactericidal but promote phagocytosis
E.   Antibodies easily destroyed by heat

1228.   SMALLPOX VACCINE:
A.   Is obtained from vaccinated horses
B.   Is prepared by making a glycerol-water suspension of vesicles of vaccinia or cowpox
C.   Must be acid to bromocresol purple
D.   Is not stable when frozen
E.   Is injected intramuscularly

1229.   RABIES VACCINE:
A.   May be stored at room temperature
B.   Provides permanent immunity
C.   Must be tested for non-infectivity in rabbits
D.   Is prepared from street virus
E.   Is prepared from serum of infected rabbits

1230.   RABIES VIRUS IS ATTENUATED BY:
A.   Drying
B.   Dilution
C.   Emulsification with phenol
D.   All of these
E.   None of these

1231.   LIVE VACCINES ARE NOT USED IN THIS COUNTRY FOR IMMUNIZATION AGAINST:
A.   Diphtheria
B.   Measles
C.   Poliomyelitis
D.   Rabies
E.   Smallpox

MATCH THE FOLLOWING DISEASES WITH CAUSATIVE AGENT:

1232. ___ Filiariasis   A. Bacteria
1233. ___ St. Louis encephalitis   B. Virus
1234. ___ Moniliasis   C. Rickettsia
1235. ___ Rocky Mountain spotted fever   D. Fungus
1236. ___ Meningitis   E. Parasite worm

1237.   NORTH AMERICAN ANTI-SNAKE BITE SERUM IS EFFECTIVE
        AGAINST THE BITE OF:
        A. Copperhead
        B. Cottonmouth moccasin
        C. Rattlesnake
        D. All of the above
        E. None of the above

1238.   RUBELLA IS ANOTHER NAME FOR:
        A. Measles
        B. Meningitis
        C. German measles
        D. Scarlet fever
        E. Mumps

1239.   THE ANTITOXIC EFFECT OF TETANUS ANTITOXIN LASTS:
        A. 4-6 hours
        B. 24 hours
        C. Indefinitely
        D. 2-3 years
        E. 10 days

1240.   IF SYMPTOMS OF TETANUS APPEAR, THE ANTITOXIN SHOULD:
        A. Be given subcutaneously
        B. Be given orally
        C. Be given intramuscularly
        D. Be given intravenously or intraspinally
        E. Not be given

1241.   BCG IS NORMALLY GIVEN:
        A. To adults by mouth
        B. To adults by injection
        C. To infants by mouth
        D. To infants by injection
        E. To anyone by injection

MATCH THE FOLLOWING:

1242. ___ Diphtheria antitoxin   A. 500 antitoxic units per cc
1243. ___ Tetanus antitoxin   B. Occurs in two types, A
1244. ___ Botulinus antitoxin   and B
                                        C. 400 antitoxic units per cc

1245.   ANTITOXINS ARE USUALLY ASSOCIATED WITH THE _____
         FRACTION OF THE BLOOD:
         A. Euglobulin   D. Leukocyte
         B. Pseudoglobulin   E. Fibrinogen
         C. Albumin

         MATCH THE FOLLOWING:

1246. ___ Atopy   A. Proteins acting as exciting agents
1247. ___ Allergen   B. Abnormal sensitization due to
1248. ___ Atoxins   proteins
                                  C. Substance which induces hyper-
                                      sensitivity

1249.   TOXINS:
         A. Are measured in terms of their M.L.D. for a certain laboratory animal
         B. Lose combining power with antitoxin before potency
         C. Are unstable when dried in vacuo
         D. Are unstable even if dried in vacuo and stored at 0° C.
         E. None of these

1250.   PERTUSSIS VACCINE U. S. P.:
         A. Is combined with diphtheria and tetanus organisms
         B. Is used for active immunization against bacterial influenza
         C. Is administered intravenously
         D. Is prepared from killed hemophilus pertussis organisms
         E. Must comply with F. D. A. regulations

         MATCH THE FOLLOWING T. B. TESTS:

1251. ___ Mantoux Test   A. Ophthalmic test
1252. ___ Von Pirquet Test   B. Percutaneous test
1253. ___ Moro Reaction   C. A cutaneous test
1254. ___ Calmette Reaction   D. Intracutaneous test
1255. ___ Patch Test   E. May be safely substituted for
                                      Mantoux Test

1256.   PERTUSSIS VACCINE:
         A. Contains a small amount of phenol or cresol as a preservative
         B. Is a detoxified suspension of hemophilus influenzae organisms
         C. Is used to passively immunize susceptible persons
         D. Consists of pertussis organisms which have been killed with 0. 5%
             phenol or 0. 4% cresol
         E. Is prepared from a strain of low antigenicity

1257.   WHICH OF THE FOLLOWING EXERTS ITS EFFECT BY INTERFERENCE
         WITH CELL WALL SYNTHESIS?
         A. Griseofulvin (Fulvicin)
         B. Nystatin (Mycostatin)
         C. Flucytosine (Ancobon)
         D. Cephalothin (Keflin)
         E. Tolnaftate (Tinactin)

1258.   POLIOMYELITIS VACCINE:
   A. Is made from type 1 and 2 strains only
   B. Should not be used if color changes
   C. May be used if turbid
   D. Should not be allowed to freeze
   E. Polio virus is killed with cresol

1259.   "BLACK DEATH" IS THE TERM ASSOCIATED WITH:
   A. Diphtheria   D. Brucellosis
   B. Whooping cough   E. Sylvatic plague
   C. Tularemia

1260.   BRUCELLOSIS IS CHARACTERIZED BY:
   A. Encephalitis   D. Rose rash
   B. Fluctuating temperature   E. Hepatitis
   C. Dysentery

1261.   P. PESTIS IS TRANSMITTED BY:
   A. Rat flea
   B. Dog bite
   C. Vaccines
   D. Fecal contamination of water
   E. Food contamination

1262.   UNDULANT FEVER IS CAUSED BY MICROORGANISMS OF THE
   _____ GENUS:
   A. Brucella   D. Scarlatina
   B. Corynebacterium   E. Hemophilus
   C. Shigella

1263.   NEGRI BODIES ARE MINUTE BODIES FOUND IN PERSONS OR ANIMALS
   INFECTED WITH:
   A. Tuberculosis   D. Typhoid fever
   B. Diphtheria   E. Rabies
   C. Scarlet fever

1264.   TULAREMIA IS TRANSMITTED BY:
   A. The bite of infected flies and ticks
   B. Mosquito bites
   C. Droplet transmission
   D. Direct contact with convalescent patients
   E. Bite of rat lice

1265.   DIPHTHERIA TOXIN EXERTS ITS TOXICITY BY:
   A. Destruction of nervous tissue
   B. Hemolysis of red cells
   C. Inactivation of respiratory enzymes
   D. Paralysis of spinal cord
   E. Damage to heart muscle

1266.   CHOLERA IS CHARACTERIZED BY:
   A. Dehydration of the tissues
   B. Bubos
   C. Erythema of the skin
   D. Dysentery
   E. Respiratory paralysis

1267.   MUMPS IN CHILDREN USUALLY INVOLVES:
        A. Salivary glands   D. Pancreas and liver
        B. Tonsils and throat   E. CNS
        C. Sex glands

1268.   GRAY PATCHES ON THE TONSILS OR MUCOUS MEMBRANE OF THE
        NOSE AND THROAT ARE ASSOCIATED WITH:
        A. Measles   D. German measles
        B. Mumps   E. Tetanus
        C. Diphtheria

1269.   THE PLAGUE:
        A. Is transmitted by the rat flea or rat louse
        B. The fleas are natural hosts
        C. Organism is never found in the tissues or exudates of those infected
        D. Immune serum is administered during infection
        E. Haffkine vaccine confers absolute immunity

1270.   TOXOIDS ARE:
        A. Obtained from culture filtrates of viable organisms
        B. Bacterial vaccines
        C. Nonspecific protein filtrates
        D. Nonantigenic toxins
        E. Unofficial toxins

1271.   KOPLIK'S SPOTS ARE ASSOCIATED WITH:
        A. Tularemia   D. Measles
        B. Rocky Mountain spotted fever   E. Scarlet fever
        C. Diphtheria

1272.   PSITTACOSIS IS DUE TO:
        A. Virus   D. Neoplasm
        B. Gram negative rod   E. Unknown
        C. Tinea cruris

1273.   WHICH ANTHELMINTHIC IS EFFECTIVE AGAINST MULTIPLE IN-
        FESTATIONS?
        A. Tolnaftate (Tinactin)
        B. Griseofulvin (Fulvicin)
        C. Tetracycline (Achromycin V)
        D. Flucytosine (Ancobon)
        E. Thiobendazole (Mintezol)

1274.   WHICH OF THE FOLLOWING DOES NOT APPLY TO S. TYPHOSA?
        A. Ferments dextrose, maltose, mannitol, without gas production
        B. Motile
        C. Gram negative
        D. Sensitive to chloromycetin
        E. Ferments lactose and sucrose with gas production

1275.   A PREVALENT RECENT TYPE OF BACTERIAL CONTAMINATION
        IN DRUGS IS FROM:
        A. Streptococcus
        B. Salmonella
        C. Influenza virus
        D. St. Louis encephalitis
        E. Rickettsia

1276.   THE PROPER INTERPRETATION OF A POSITIVE REACTION TO A
        TUBERCULIN TEST IS THAT THE PERSON IS:
        A. Suffering from active tuberculosis
        B. Immune to invasion by the tubercle bacillus
        C. Susceptible to invasion by the tubercle bacillus
        D. Sensitive to tuberculo-protein by virtue of previous or present
            infection with tubercle bacillus
        E. None of the above

1277.   ATHLETE'S FOOT IS CAUSED BY:
        A. Bacteria
        B. Viruses
        C. Rickettsia
        D. Parasitic worms
        E. Fungi

1278.   PERTUSSIS VACCINE IS ADMINISTERED:
        A. Subcutaneously in 3 to 5 doses
        B. Hypodermically in 0.5 cc. and 0.1 cc. doses
        C. Hypodermically in a total dose of 60,000
        D. In 3 individual doses of 0.1 cc. each
        E. In a single intravenous dose

1279.   HEMOLYTIC STREPTOCOCCI ARE CLASSIFIED ON THE BASIS OF:
        A. C reactive protein   D. VW complex
        B. A carbohydrate and M protein   E. Dye tolerance
        C. H, O and Vi antigens

1280.   THE SABIN VACCINE IS SUPERIOR TO SALK VACCINE BECAUSE:
        A. It imparts permanent immunity
        B. It is genetically unstable
        C. It can be administered orally
        D. It requires fewer injections
        E. It is more readily available

1281.   BY AN OXIDATIVE ENZYME IS MEANT AN ENZYME WHICH:
        A. Activates hydrogen to combine with the substrate
        B. Splits off amino groups
        C. Activates oxygen to combine with substrate
        D. Brings about mutations
        E. Hydrolyzes carbohydrates

1282.   COUPLED WITH THE STEPWISE TRANSPORT OF ELECTRONS FROM
        VARIOUS OXIDIZABLE SUBSTANCES TO OXYGEN, IS A MOST IMPORT-
        ANT CELLULAR PROCESS CALLED:
        A. Alcoholic fermentation
        B. Formation of co-enzymes
        C. Oxidative phosphorylation
        D. Transamination
        E. Hydrogenation

1283. STREPTOCOCCUS VIRIDANS IS ASSOCIATED WITH:
A. Myositis, cystitis, arthritis
B. Pyorrhea alveolaris, subacute bacterial endocarditis, urinary tract
       infection
C. Scarlet fever, erysipelas, septic sore throat
D. Meningitis, arthritis, conjunctivitis
E. Furunculosis, carbuncle, lung abscess

1284. THE ONLY RECOGNIZED RESERVOIR OF MENINGOCOCCUS IS:
A. Sheep   D. Man
B. Infected swine   E. Household pets
C. Rodents

1285. THE ANIMAL RESERVOIRS OF TULAREMIA IN THE U.S. ARE CHIEFLY:
A. Rodents, semi-aquatic mammals and sheep
B. Dogs and other canines
C. House pets
D. Fowl and game birds
E. Mites and ticks

1286. DRUG FASTNESS MAY BE PRODUCED IF:
A. Microorganisms are acid fast
B. Microorganisms are grown on blood agar
C. Microorganisms are kept in contact with small sublethal concentra-
       tions of drug
D. Frequent large doses of drug are added
E. None of these

1287. THE RATE OF GROWTH OF MYCOBACTERIA:
A. Is rapid but faster under anaerobic conditions
B. Is inhibited by 10% CO_2
C. Is independent of growth factors
D. Is among the slowest for all bacteria
E. Is optimal at pH 8

1288. THE TIME OF DAY WHEN FEVERS TEND TO PEAK IS _____.
A. 2 to 4 p.m.
B. 4 to 6 p.m.
C. 6 to 10 p.m.
D. 10 to 12 p.m.
E. 10 to 12 a.m.

1289. PHENOL COEFFICIENT INDICATES:
A. Concentration of disinfectant in solution
B. Effectiveness of tested disinfectant as compared to pure phenol
C. Highest dilution of X not killing organisms in five minutes but killing
       in ten minutes
D. Amount of irritation to body tissues
E. Increase in cellular growth

1290. THE OPTIMAL AND LIMITING TEMPERATURES FOR BACTERIA:
A. Are same for all bacteria
B. Are optimal and limiting temperatures of their enzymes
C. Are ranges within which spore formation occurs
D. Are ranges within which anaerobic bacteria grow best
E. None of these

1291.   THE GENUS CLOSTRIDIUM ARE NOTED FOR ALL BEING:
        A. Normally harmless GI saprophytes
        B. Spore-forming rods dependent to a greater or lesser degree on
            anaerobiosis
        C. Motile by bipolar flagella
        D. Possessing a capsule composed of D-galactose polymer
        E. Neurotoxic

1292.   TYPHUS IS CAUSED BY:
        A. Rickettsia
        B. Viruses
        C. Bacteria
        D. Molds or yeasts
        E. None of the above

1293.   GRAM POSITIVE BACTERIA, AFTER BEING STAINED WITH A
        COUNTERSTAIN ARE:
        A. Yellow   D. Violet
        B. Orange   E. Green
        C. Red

1294.   A MORDANT IS USED AS:
        A. An agent inducing death
        B. A decolorizing solution for acid fast organisms
        C. A substance that fixes bacterial stain so the material will retain it
        D. Selective stain for capsules
        E. None of these

1295.   ENZYMES ARE CLASSIFIED ON THE BASIS OF:
        A. Their structure
        B. Their chemical composition
        C. Substrate acted upon by them
        D. Where they are found in human body
        E. All are correct

1296.   IN ORDER TO KILL SPORES:
        A. Autoclave for 15-20 minutes at 120 degrees Centigrade
        B. Steam the media for 15-20 minutes
        C. Raise temperature slowly to 90 degrees Centigrade and maintain this
            temperature for one hour
        D. Heat 15-30 minutes at 100 degrees Centigrade in moist heat on 3
            successive days
        E. A and B are both correct

1297.   THE TYPE OF MEDIUM USED TO STUDY COLONY CHARACTERISTICS:
        A. Meat infusion broth   D. Infusion agar plate
        B. Gelatin plate   E. Surface agar plate
        C. Agar slant

1298.   THE INCUBATION PERIOD OF RABIES IN MAN IS_____.
        A. Two to four weeks
        B. One to three weeks
        C. One to two months
        D. Up to one year
        E. Up to two years or more

1299.   THE WORD ANTIBIOTIC MEANS:
    A.   Bacteriological enzyme
    B.   Antigrowth substance
    C.   Bacteriostatic substance produced by micro-organisms
    D.   Both A and B are correct
    E.   Both B and C are correct

1300.   WHICH ONE OF THE FOLLOWING NEVER POSSESSES A CAPSULE?
    A.   D. Pneumoniae
    B.   H. Influenzae
    C.   B. Anthracis
    D.   Strep. Pyogenes
    E.   C. Diphtheriae

1301.   WHICH OF THE FOLLOWING IS NOT AN INTEGRAL PART OF THE
    GROWTH SEQUENCE OF A BACTERIAL COLONY?
    A.   Lag phase   D.   Sporulation phase
    B.   Acceleration phase   E.   Death phase
    C.   Exponential phase

1302.   A DISEASE NOT PRODUCED BY A VIRUS IS:
    A.   Septic sore throat   D.   Mumps
    B.   Smallpox   E.   Yellow fever
    C.   Rabies

1303.   THE ORGANISM MOST FREQUENTLY RESPONSIBLE FOR SALMONELLA
    GASTROENTERITIS IS:
    A.   Salmonella Hirschfeldii   D.   Salmonella Typhimurium
    B.   Salmonella Choleraesuis   E.   Salmonella Newport
    C.   Salmonella Schottmüelleri

1304.   WHICH OF THE FOLLOWING MEN IS CREDITED WITH FIRST
    PROPAGATING THE VIRUS OF POLIO?
    A.   Cox   D.   Salk
    B.   Enders   E.   Sabin
    C.   Koprowski

1305.   SHIGELLA ARE USUALLY CLASSIFIED BY:
    A.   Fermentation reactions   D.   Phage typing
    B.   Antigenic characters   E.   Dye tolerance
    C.   Combination of A and B

1306.   A RICKETTSIAL DISEASE WHICH CAN BECOME AN EPIDEMIC
    THROUGH INFECTED LICE IS:
    A.   Typhoid
    B.   Poliomyelitis
    C.   Scarlet fever
    D.   Typhus
    E.   Chickenpox

1307.   WHAT ARE THE PROPERTIES HEMOPHILUS INFLUENZAE AND
        NEISSERIA INTRACELLULARIS HAVE IN COMMON?
        A. Both cause infection of inner ear
        B. Both are strict parasites on man and cause meningitis
        C. Both are bacilli and stain acid fast
        D. Both produce capsules
        E. There are no common properties

1308.   ALL OF THE FOLLOWING CHARACTERIZE PASTEURELLA
        EXCEPT:
        A. Gram negative, bipolar staining ovoid rods
        B. Mainly parasitic on animals, man secondarily infected
        C. Obligate anaerobes
        D. Liquefaction of gelatin
        E. Fermentation of carbohydrates with acid but no gas

1309.   MOST FOOD POISONING IS CAUSED BY SPECIES OF:
        A. Typhus
        B. Salmonella
        C. Shigella
        D. Tetanus
        E. Pasteurella

1310.   PRIMARY CULTIVATION OF GONOCOCCUS ON LABORATORY MEDIA
        IS DIFFICULT BECAUSE:
        A. The coccus can survive only in living tissues
        B. It is susceptible to the toxic effect of substances commonly present
            in media
        C. Autolysis occurs
        D. Of the presence of glutamine
        E. No suitable medium has yet been found

1311.   THE TREATMENT OF CHOICE FOR LEPROSY IS_____.
        A. Penicillin therapy   D. Sulfone therapy
        B. Broad spectrum antibiotic therapy   E. None of these
        C. Chloromycetin therapy

1312.   WHICH SYMPTOM IS NOT TYPICAL OF GRAM NEGATIVE BACTEREMIA?
        A. Marked leukocytosis   D. Polyuria
        B. High fever   E. Hypotension
        C. Abrupt onset of chills

1313.   IN THE COURSE OF AN ATTACK OF DYSENTERY, THE ORGANISM IS
        BEST RECOVERED FROM:
        A. The blood stream at peak of fever
        B. Biopsy of rectal mucosa
        C. The stool mucus
        D. The urine
        E. The saliva

1314. ANTIGEN IS:
       A. Any foreign material introduced into the human body
       B. Only protein in nature
       C. Contained in serum injected in vaccination
       D. Any protein and few microbiological polysaccharides that when
           injected stimulate production of antibodies against themselves
       E. All of the above are correct

1315. ONE OF THE FOLLOWING IS NOT A CLASSIFICATION OF VIRUSES:
       A. Dermatropic   D. Neoplastic
       B. Neurotropic   E. Somatophilic
       C. Viscerotropic

1316. THE FIRST STEP IN OBTAINING A PURE CULTURE OF ANY BACTERIA
       IS:
       A. Incubation of the test organism in beef broth
       B. Streak a droplet of the specimen on an agar plate and incubate
       C. Spread a droplet on ss agar
       D. Plate the bacteria out on gelatin
       E. Any of these

1317. WHICH OF THE FOLLOWING IS NOT PRODUCED BY MOLDS?
       A. Penicillin   D. Bacitracin
       B. Terramycin   E. Neomycin
       C. Streptomycin

1318. AN ADVANTAGE IN THE USE OF SYNTHETIC MEDIA IS:
       A. Their reproducibility
       B. Absence of proteins in media
       C. Absence of antigenic or allergic properties when injected into man
       D. Their exactly known composition
       E. All the statements are true

1319. YELLOW FEVER IS:
       A. Transmitted by the body and head louse
       B. Found mainly in temperate climates
       C. Transmitted by the female Anopheles mosquito
       D. Capable of causing a viral disease in epidemic proportions
       E. Prevented by means of a vaccine extremely stable to heat and light

1320. THE MICROORGANISM VIBRIO COMMA CAUSES:
       A. Rat bite fever
       B. Scarlet fever
       C. Cholera
       D. Mumps
       E. Rocky Mountain spotted fever

1321.   AGGLUTININS ARE:
A. Antitoxins which lyse bacteria
B. Carbohydrates
C. A product of bacterial secretions
D. Antibodies which cause bacteria to clump together
E. Nonspecific

1322.   BY STERILIZATION IS MEANT:
A. Freeing an object from life of any kind
B. Removal of organisms capable of causing infection
C. Inhibition of growth of bacteria
D. Removal of facultative anaerobes
E. None of these

1323.   DRUG FASTNESS MAY BE ATTRIBUTED TO:
A. Inferior quality of drug
B. Chemical changes of the drug brought about by the bacteria
C. Mutant forms of the original bacterial strain
D. Use of wrong drug
E. None of these

1324.   PROTEUS VULGARIS MAY BE DISTINGUISHED ON PLATE CULTURE
FROM MOST OTHER ENTERIC BACTERIA BY THE PRESENCE OF:
A. Formation of blue pigment   D. Swarming
B. Hemolysis   E. Liquefaction of agar
C. Action on lactose

1325.   BACTERIAL CELLS THAT EXHIBIT ACID FAST PROPERTIES DIFFER
FROM OTHER BACTERIAL CELLS BY:
A. Containing nucleoproteins
B. They do not differ chemically
C. High concentration of fatty acids
D. Presence of mycolic acid in combination with waxy material
E. Both C and D are correct

1326.   THE ACTION OF CLOSTRIDIUM BOTULINUM IN DISEASE IS DUE TO:
A. Number of living bacteria
B. Presence of clostridium in intestines
C. Exotoxin ingested
D. Endotoxins produced
E. Statements A and B are both correct

1327.   VIRUSES AND RICKETTSIAE DIFFER FROM BACTERIA IN THEIR
FOOD REQUIREMENTS BECAUSE:
A. They can only live on synthetic media
B. They can only multiply in the presence of bacteria
C. They need sunlight for growth
D. They cannot survive without the presence of living tissue
E. They can only grow in soil

1328.   _____ IS USUALLY ASSOCIATED WITH HIGH INCIDENCE OF
CONCOMITANT PRE-MENINGITIS.
A. Peritonsillar abscess   D. Cervical adenitis
B. Otitis media   E. Pneumonitis
C. Quinsy

1329.   WHICH OF THE FOLLOWING SUBSTANCES IS USED TO TEST THE
ACIDITY OF A CULTURE MEDIUM?
A. Lead acetate paper   D. Indicator
B. Iodine   E. Either A or B is correct
C. Nucleic acid

1330.   SECOND ATTACKS OF SCARLET FEVER ARE RARE BECAUSE:
A. Antibodies to the erythrogenic toxin prevent the recurrence of the
    skin rash even in the event of a second streptococcal infection
B. One attack confers permanent immunity to Strep. Scarlatinae though
    the patient is susceptible to other strains
C. The causative agent of the rash remains permanently attached to the
    skin and organs and prevents the response
D. The reason is unknown, but it is an empirical clinical fact
E. None of these

1331.   REACTIONS OF ANTIGENS WITH ANTIBODIES ARE:
A. Slow   D. Controlled by temperature
B. Rare   E. Highly specific
C. Impossible

1332.   THERMAL DEATH POINT:
A. All bacteria of a given species are killed after 10 minutes exposure
B. All bacteria of a given species are killed after 20 minutes exposure
C. All bacteria are killed instantaneously
D. Half of the virulent organisms are killed
E. Lysis of bacteria begins

1333.   TETANUS TOXIN IS NOW KNOWN TO BE A (AN):
A. Protein   D. Anticholinesterase
B. Carbohydrate   E. Amine oxidase inhibitor
C. Hapten

1334.   UNDULANT FEVER IS USUALLY TRANSMITTED BY:
A. Humans
B. Insect vectors
C. Food or milk
D. Sneezing
E. Mice

1335.   UNDULANT FEVER IS SYNONYMOUS WITH:
A. Bubonic plague
B. Cholera
C. Brucellosis
D. Pneumonia
E. Splenic fever

1336.   METRONIDAZOLE IS USED MAINLY TO TREAT:
A. Resistant staph
B. Syphilis
C. Gonorrhea
D. Trichomonas
E. Pneumonia

1337.   THE DICK REACTION IS:
A. A complement fixation reaction
B. The same as the Arthus phenomenon
C. An erythrogenic toxin reaction
D. Caused by hypersensitivity to antitoxin
E. An immune reaction

1338.   TRENCH MOUTH IS CAUSED BY:
A. B. vincentii
B. Leptospira
C. S. aureus
D. E. coli
E. None of these

1339.   ENTEROCOCCI ARE:
A. Commonly found in human and animal intestines
B. Never pathogenic
C. The etiological agents of typhoid fever
D. The cause of scarlet fever
E. Found in the erythrocytes
F. Motile

1340.   PARALYTIC POLIO:
A. Is more common in temperate than tropical zone
B. Can be readily cured
C. Is no longer seen
D. Is more common now than 5 years ago
E. Is caused by a bacteria

IN THE FOLLOWING DISEASES, THE CLINICAL MANIFESTATIONS
ARE CAUSED BY:

1341. ___ Tetanus   A. Endotoxin
1342. ___ Botulism   B. Exotoxin
1343. ___ Typhoid
1344. ___ Diphtheria

1345.   AUTOGENOUS VACCINES ARE:
A. Vaccines prepared from autotrophic bacteria
B. Prepared from autolytic organisms
C. Prepared from patient's own organisms
D. Identical with stock vaccines
E. Administered for passive immunization

1346. BACTERIAL ANTIGENS ARE:
A. Vectors of disease
B. Antibiotic substances
C. May be demonstrated in the specific antibacterial serum
D. Used to produce active immunity
E. Never produce disease

1347. ONE OF KOCH'S POSTULATES IS TO:
A. Demonstrate the etiological agent of a disease
B. Illustrate specific hypersensitivity
C. Demonstrate the mode of transmission
D. Determine the organism serologically
E. Determine specific phagocyte agents

1348. THE REAGENT USED TO DETERMINE SUSCEPTIBILITY TO
DIPHTHERIA IS:
A. Toxoid
B. Culture of diphtheria organisms
C. Diphtheria antitoxin
D. Alum-precipitated toxoid
E. Diphtheria toxin unmodified

1349. ACTIVE IMMUNIZATION AGAINST DIPHTHERIA MAY BE DEVELOPED
BY INJECTIONS WITH:
A. Alum-precipitated culture
B. Antitoxin
C. Filtrates of C. Hoffmanni and C. Xerosis cultures
D. Toxoid
E. Antidiphtheritic serum

1350. THE DEVELOPMENT OF ANAEROBIC BACTERIA IN A MEDIUM
CONTAINING AEROBIC ORGANISMS IS AN EXAMPLE OF:
A. Parasitism   D. Synergism
B. Commensalism   E. Satellitism
C. Symbiosis

1351. IN YOUNG CHILDREN TETRACYCLINES OFTEN CAUSE:
A. Agranulocytosis   D. Muscular weakness
B. Discoloration of teeth E. Hyperplasia of the gums
C. Conjunctivitis

1352. THE ETIOLOGIC AGENT OF MONONUCLEOSIS IS:
A. Epstein-Barr virus
B. Beta-hemolytic streptococcus
C. Resistant staphylococcus
D. A Rickettsia
E. A fungus

1353.   DIPHTHERIA TOXIN:
A.   Is obtained from fluid extracts of the culture
B.   Contains the avirulent organisms suspended in saline
C.   Is obtained from the blood serum of an immunized horse
D.   Is a mixed culture filtrate of the pathogenic strains of C. Diphtheriae
E.   Is obtained from chick embryo cultures

1354.   AN ADVANTAGE OF IODOPHORS OVER IODINE SOLUTIONS IS:
A.   Increased antiseptic activity
B.   Easier to apply
C.   Do not stain
D.   Cause less pain on wounds
E.   None of these

1355.   PASSIVE IMMUNITY IS THE RESULT OF:
A.   Injection with the specific antigen
B.   Injection with the specific antibody
C.   A lack of response to the antigen
D.   Partial immunization
E.   Recovery from a specific infection

1356.   IMMUNIZATION AGAINST MEASLES EMPLOYS:
A.   A measles toxoid
B.   Gamma globulin
C.   A live virus
D.   Live bacteria
E.   Attenuated virus

1357.   WHICH IS MOST EFFECTIVE TO TREAT TYPHOID?
A.   Tetracyclines
B.   Penicillin G
C.   Erythromycin
D.   Sulfonamides
E.   Ampicillin

1358.   BETA HEMOLYSIS:
A.   Causes dissolution of the phagocytes
B.   Cannot be demonstrated in the absence of complement
C.   Is characteristic of D. pneumoniae
D.   Is characteristic of scarlet fever strains of streptococci
E.   Is best demonstrated on chocolate agar plates

1359.   INTERFERON IS:
A.   An enzyme
B.   A protein complex
C.   An agglutinogen
D.   A precursor of amino acids
E.   None of these

1360.   THE INCUBATION PERIOD FOR MUMPS IN HUMANS IS USUALLY:
A.   14 to 21 days
B.   7 to 14 days
C.   1 to 7 days
D.   15 to 28 days
E.   21 to 30 days

1361.   WHICH OF THE FOLLOWING IS USED SPECIFICALLY TO TREAT
        GONORRHEA?
        A. Novobiocin   D. Cycloserine
        B. Spectinomycin   E. Cephazolin
        C. Viomycin

1362.   YELLOW FEVER VACCINE:
        A. Is quite stable
        B. Must be used within 1/2 hour after reconstitution
        C. Is very stable under refrigeration
        D. Given on 3 consecutive days
        E. Is not used any longer

MATCH THE FOLLOWING:

1363. ___ Streptococcus Scarlatinae   A. Plague
1364. ___ Mycobacterium Leprae   B. Scarlet fever
1365. ___ Pasteurella Pestis   C. Whooping cough
1366. ___ Hemophilus Pertussis   D. Gas gangrene
1367. ___ Clostridium Perfringens   E. Hansen's disease

MATCH THE FOLLOWING:

1368. ___ Treponema Pallidum   A. Infectious jaundice
1369. ___ Leptospira Ictero Hemorrhagica   B. Typhus
1370. ___ Rickettsia Prowazeki   C. Malaria
1371. ___ Hemophilus Ducreyi   D. Syphilis
1372. ___ Plasmodium Vivax   E. Chancroid

MATCH THE DRUG OF CHOICE WITH THE DISEASE OR CONDTION:

1373. ___ Chloromycetin   A. Undiagnosed sepsis
1374. ___ Pyrvinium pamoate   B. Elephantiasis
1375. ___ Quinacrine   C. Typhoid fever
1376. ___ Ampicillin   D. Pinworm infestations
1377. ___ Garamycin   E. Tapeworm infestations

MATCH THE FOLLOWING:

1378. ___ Rickets   A. Protozoal disease
1379. ___ Chaga's disease   B. Mycotic disease
1380. ___ Amebiasis   C. Viral disease
1381. ___ Blastomycosis   D. Streptococcal
1382. ___ Dengue fever   E. Non-infectious disease
1383. ___ Erysipelas

1384.   PATHOGENIC STAPHYLOCOCCI IN CARRIERS ARE USUALLY
        HARBORED IN:
        A. Nose and skin
        B. Gastrointestinal tract
        C. Kidney and bladder
        D. Salivary glands
        E. All of these

1385.   AN ORGAN OF THE BODY THAT IS OFTEN DAMAGED PER-
        MANENTLY BY RHEUMATIC FEVER IS THE:
        A. Lung   D. Liver
        B. Kidney   E. Spleen
        C. Heart

1386.   A VARIETY OF STAPH. AUREUS THAT IS VERY RESISTANT TO
        HEAT IS:
        A. Caloris   D. Lactophilus
        B. Communis   E. Globigii
        C. Thermophilus

1387.   HUMAN DISEASE THAT CAN BE TRANSMITTED BY MILK IS
        CAUSED BY:
        A. Streptococcus lactis   D. Aerobacter aerogenes
        B. Bacillus anthracis   E. Streptococcus aglatinae
        C. Streptococcus epidemicus

1388.   GAS GANGRENE IS COMMONLY CAUSED BY:
        A. Pasteurella   D. Shigella
        B. Clostridia   E. Mycobacteria
        C. Rickettsia

1389.   _____ IS ANY PUS-FORMING SKIN INFECTION.
        A. Dermatitis
        B. Empyema
        C. Emphysema
        D. Pyoderma
        E. Coryza

1390.   THE ORGANISM CAUSING URINARY TRACT INFECTIONS IS:
        A. E. coli   D. Staphylococcus pyogenes
        B. Proteus vulgaris   E. All of these
        C. Pseudomonas aeruginosa

1391.   DARK FIELD ILLUMINATION IS USED IN CASES WHERE:
        A. Bacteria are difficult to stain
        B. Living bacteria are to be studied
        C. Presence of cytoplasmic granules is to be determined
        D. Main object of the study is cell wall
        E. A and B are both correct

1392.   THE MECHANISM OF DRY HEAT STERILIZATION IS PRIMARILY:
        A. Oxidation
        B. Reduction
        C. Coagulation
        D. Denaturation
        E. None of the above

1393.   BACILLARY DYSENTERY IS USUALLY CAUSED BY_____
        ORGANISMS:
        A. Pasteurella
        B. E. Coli
        C. Shigella
        D. Plasmodium
        E. Ascaria

1394.   UNTREATED GONORRHEA IN THE FEMALE MAY CAUSE:
         A. Discoloration of teeth
         B. Abortion
         C. Increased incidence of carcinoma
         D. Sterility
         E. Fungal infections

1395.   THE PREFERRED METHOD OF STERILIZATION FOR MINERAL OIL IS:
         A. Autoclave   D. Dry heat
         B. Bacterial filtration   E. Radiation
         C. Gas sterilization

1396.   _____ SHOULD BE USED FOR SEVERE POTENTIALLY FATAL
         FUNGAL INFECTIONS.
         A. Nystatin
         B. Griseofulvin
         C. Amphotericin B
         D. Candidicin
         E. Gentian violet

1397.   THRUSH IS CAUSED BY A (AN):
         A. Rickettsia
         B. Streptococcus
         C. Staphylococcus
         D. Fungus
         E. Virus

1398.   ALL BUT ONE OF THE FOLLOWING "TOXINS" ARE TYPICAL OF ALL
         PATHOGENIC STAPHYLOCOCCI:
         A. Hemolysin   D. Coagulase
         B. Leukocidin   E. Fibrinolysin
         C. Enterotoxin

1399.   BACTERIOPHAGES ARE USUALLY:
         A. Bacteria   D. Polysaccharides
         B. Viruses   E. None of these
         C. Lipoidal

1400.   WEIL-FELIX REACTION IS A TEST FOR:
         A. Typhus fever
         B. Malaria
         C. Yellow fever
         D. Presence of Clostridium botulinum
         E. None of the above

1401.   HISTOPLASMOSIS IS BEST TREATED WITH:
         A. Penicillin G
         B. Amphotericin B
         C. Ampicillin
         D. Tetracycline
         E. Garamycin

1402. AN ANTIBODY IS CHEMICALLY:
A. A protein
B. A polysaccharide
C. An amino acid
D. Any foreign substance in the body
E. None of these

1403. THE BASIC TYPES OF FOOD FOR MICROORGANISMS ARE:
A. Glucose, amino acids and inorganic substances
B. Blood cells and lymph
C. Only obtained from the soil
D. Found in chick embryos
E. Carbon and hydrogen

1404. SCABIES IS A DISEASE OF THE:
A. Mouth
B. Skin
C. Liver
D. Lungs
E. G.I. tract

1405. THE MOST EFFECTIVE DRUGS AGAINST PROTEUS SPECIES ARE:
A. Penicillins   D. Nitrofurantoins
B. Sulfonamides   E. Erythromycins
C. Tetracyclines

1406. TYNDALLIZATION IS ALSO CALLED:
A. Filtration
B. Gas sterilization
C. Fractional sterilization
D. Pasteurization
E. Ionization by radiation

1407. ROCKY MOUNTAIN SPOTTED FEVER IS CAUSED BY_____.
A. A virus
B. A rickettsia
C. A bacteria
D. An amoeba
E. None of the above

1408. PENICILLIN G HAS WEAKEST BACTERIOSTATIC EFFECT
AGAINST:
A. Gram positive bacilli   D. Neisseria species
B. Gram negative bacilli   E. B and D are correct
C. Micrococci

1409. ETHYLENE OXIDE STERILIZES BY A MECHANISM PRIMARILY
INVOLVING:
A. Coagulation
B. Oxidation
C. Alkylation
D. Hydrolysis
E. Denaturation

1410.   A PATHOGENIC FUNGUS IS:
A.   Trichoderma viride
B.   Rhizopus nigricans
C.   Geotrichum candium
D.   Blastomyces dermatitidis
E.   C and D are correct

1411.   ANTISEPTIC IS DEFINED AS:
A.   A solution that kills bacteria
B.   A chemical substance that inhibits all microorganisms
C.   A substance that inhibits bacteria after being absorbed into the
circulation
D.   A substance that retards or inhibits growth of infectious agents
E.   All are correct

1412.   MYCOBACTERIA ARE INDEPENDENT OF ALL VITAMINS, EXCEPT:
A.   Vitamin B_1 D.   Vitamin B_{12}
B.   Vitamin B_2 E.   Biotin
C.   Vitamin B_6

1413.   AN ANTIBIOTIC OF THERAPEUTIC VALUE IS PRODUCED BY:
A.   Penicillium roqueforti   D.   Aspergillum glaucus
B.   Penicillium chrysogenum   E.   Penicillium italicum
C.   Streptomyces scabies

1414.   WHICH OF THE FOLLOWING ORGANISMS IS CAPABLE OF DEVITALI-
ZING LIVING TISSUE IN GAS GANGRENE?
A.   Cl. welchii   D.   Cl. sporogenes
B.   Cl. novyii   E.   Cl. histolyticum
C.   Cl. septicum

1415.   GENTAMICIN CLOSELY RESEMBLES:
A.   Novobiocin
B.   Kanamycin
C.   Penicillin G
D.   Lincomycin
E.   Polymyxin B

1416.   BACITRACIN CAN BE OBTAINED FROM A STRAIN OF:
A.   E. Coli
B.   P. aeruginosa
C.   B. subtilis
D.   S. Aureus
E.   None of the above

1417.   THE INTERMEDIATE HOST FOR SCHISTOSOMIASIS IS A:
A.   Dog
B.   Snail
C.   Flea
D.   Bird
E.   Mosquito

1418.   THE FUNCTION OF ANTIBODIES IN IMMUNITY IS:
A.   To neutralize toxins
B.   Entirely bacteriostatic
C.   To produce more leukocytes
D.   To build up resistance against any infection
E.   A and D are correct

1419.   THE BEST WAY TO CONTROL MUMPS IS WITH:
A.   Immune Globulin   D.   Sulfonamides
B.   Penicillin   E.   None of these
C.   Prophylactic vaccine

1420.   WHICH IS BEST TO TREAT RINGWORM OF THE BODY?
A.   Boric acid
B.   Tolnaftate
C.   Penicillin V
D.   Gentamycin
E.   Iodoform

1421.   A TEST USED TO CHECK LEAKAGE OF BACTERIAL FILTERS IS:
A.   The Seitz test   D.   Bubble point
B.   The millipore test   E.   None of these
C.   The seep test

1422.   VANCOMYCIN IS EFFECTIVE PRIMARILY AGAINST:
A.   Gram-positive bacilli
B.   Gram-negative bacilli
C.   Gram-positive cocci
D.   Gram-negative cocci
E.   Encapsulated forms

1423.   RHEUMATIC FEVER IS USUALLY PRECIPITATED BY:
A.   Virus infections
B.   Staph infections
C.   Mycotic infestations
D.   Streptococcal infections
E.   None of the above

1424.   PENICILLINASES ARE:
A.   Antibiotics
B.   A crude form of penicillin
C.   Enzymes which destroy penicillin
D.   Broths from which penicillin has been extracted
E.   Substance present in all penicillin susceptible to strains of
      micrococci

1425.   THE MOST COMMON LOCATION OF THE ORGANISMS IN A
        TYPHOID CARRIER IS:
        A. Nasopharynx
        B. Gallbladder
        C. Epididymis or fallopian tube
        D. Kidney
        E. Large bowel and nodes of gut

1426.   SHIGELLA ARE DIVIDED INTO "SHIGELLA DYSENTERIAE" AND
        "SHIGELLA PARADYSENTERIAE" GROUPS BY THE ABILITY TO:
        A. Ferment mannitol
        B. Ferment sorbitol
        C. Ferment lactose
        D. Ferment inositol
        E. Produce indole

1427.   PASSIVE IMMUNITY USUALLY GIVES _____ PROTECTION
        TO THE PATIENT:
        A. No
        B. Complete
        C. Long term
        D. Short term
        E. Undetermined

1428.   THE ETIOLOGICAL AGENT OF RABIES IS:
        A. A bacteria
        B. A virus
        C. A fungus
        D. A mold
        E. A rickettsia

1429.   HEPA FILTERS ARE WIDELY USED IN:
        A. Autoclaves
        B. Laminar flow hoods
        C. Face masks
        D. Oxygen masks
        E. Gas sterilizers

1430.   CEPHALOSPORINS ARE:
        A. Vaccines   D. Serums
        B. Diagnostic test agents   E. Antigens
        C. Antibiotics

1431.   HOOKWORM IS CAUSED BY:
        A. Ancylostoma duodenale
        B. Plasmodium vivax
        C. Salmonella typhosa
        D. Endamoeba histolytica
        E. Trichinella spiralis

1432.   THE ONLY FILTRABLE RICKETTSIA IS THE ONE CAUSING:
         A. Scrub typhus   D. Q fever
         B. Rocky Mountain spotted fever   E. Tick-bite fever
         C. Typhus

1433.   VIBRIO COMMA IS THE CAUSATIVE AGENT OF:
         A. Yellow fever   D. Asiatic cholera
         B. Brucellosis   E. Mumps
         C. Gonorrhea

1434.   A BACTERIOSTATIC AGENT HAS THE FOLLOWING EFFECT ON
         BACTERIA:
         A. It kills bacteria on contact
         B. It enhances their growth
         C. It induces spore formation
         D. It inhibits multiplication of bacteria
         E. It dehydrates the bacteria

1435.   AN ANAPHYLACTIC REACTION IS AN INDICATION OF:
         A. No antibodies are present in blood
         B. Immunity
         C. Hypersensitivity to given protein
         D. Presence of typhoid bacilli
         E. Infestation by Trypanosomes

1436.   TETANUS TOXIN PRODUCES THE FOLLOWING DISTINGUISHING
         EFFECT IN ITS HUMAN HOST:
         A. Gas gangrene
         B. Disturbance of vision
         C. Paralysis of throat muscles
         D. Continuous contraction of the muscles
         E. Dysentery

1437.   SCARLET FEVER IS USUALLY TREATED WITH:
         A. Sulfa drugs   D. Tetracycline
         B. Penicillin   E. Streptomycin
         C. Chloramphenicol

1438.   PENICILLINS CAN BE OBTAINED COMMERCIALLY FROM:
         A. Yeasts
         B. Molds
         C. Animal sources
         D. Fungi
         E. Bacteria

1439.   ALL OF THE FOLLOWING MAY BE PRODUCED BY CLOSTRIDIA,
         EXCEPT:
         A. Food intoxication
         B. Food poisoning
         C. Wound infection
         D. Myositis
         E. Pneumonia

1440. THE MOST IMPORTANT SINGLE STEP IN TREATING GAS GANGRENE
IS:
A. Specific antitoxin
B. Adequate surgical removal of devitalized tissue
C. Systemic antibodies
D. Fever therapy
E. Local antibiotic therapy

1441. THE MODE OF SPREAD OF BOTULINUM TOXIN IN THE BODY IS BY:
A. Direct extension along nerve trunks
B. Blood stream spread
C. Lymphatic spread
D. Direct contiguity in the gut wall
E. All are correct

1442. A SKIN DISEASE WHICH OCCURS IN BOTH NODULAR,CUTANEOUS AND
NEURAL ANESTHETIC FORMS IS:
A. Granuloma inguinale   D. Leprosy
B. Rickettsial pox   E. Pinta
C. Yaws

1443. EPIDEMIC PAROTITIS IS MORE COMMONLY CALLED:
A. Flu
B. St. Louis encephalitis
C. Common cold
D. Mumps
E. Measles

1444. BOTULISM TOXIN:
A. Is frequently found in meats
B. Comes from an organism found commonly in soil
C. Grows well in an acid medium
D. All of the above
E. None of the above

1445. SPECIES OF PROTEUS ARE IMPLICATED IN:
A. Wound infections   D. Gastroenteritis
B. Urinary tract infections   E. All are correct
C. Peritonitis

1446. THE DISEASE VARICELLA IS COMMONLY KNOWN AS:
A. Smallpox   D. Scarlet fever
B. Measles   E. Chickenpox
C. Mononucleosis

1447. A FOMITE IS:
A. An airborne carrier of disease
B. An inanimate object which transmits disease
C. A symptom of throat infections
D. A means of preventing disease
E. A type of immunity

1448.   ALTHOUGH NORMALLY A HARMLESS SAPROPHYTE, E. COLI IS THE
        MOST COMMON SOURCE OF:
        A. Peritonitis   D. Pancreatitis
        B. Cholecystitis   E. Appendicitis
        C. Acute genitourinary infections

1449.   THE MAJOR DIFFERENCE BETWEEN THE ALPHA AND BETA
        STAPHYLOCOCCAL HEMOLYSINS IS:
        A. Human erythrocytes are resistant to alpha but destroyed by beta
        B. Human erythrocytes are destroyed by alpha but not by beta
        C. Sheep RBC's are destroyed by beta but are resistant to alpha
        D. Rabbit RBC's are most susceptible of all to alpha but resistant to beta
        E. The toxins must be distinguished antigenically

1450.   THE VIRULENCE OF A STRAIN OF PNEUMOCOCCI IS RELATED TO:
        A. Their quellung reaction
        B. H antigen
        C. Vi antigen
        D. S-R variation
        E. Ability to ferment inulin

1451.   THE USUAL INCUBATION PERIOD FOR SCARLET FEVER IS:
        A. 1 to 3 days   D. 12 to 21 days
        B. 2 to 5 days   E. 14 to 24 days
        C. 8 to 13 days

1452.   A ZONE PHENOMENON IS OBTAINED:
        A. When optimal relative proportions of antigen and antibody are used
            in reaction
        B. When unequal amounts of antigen and antibody are used
        C. When a visible precipitate occurs in an antigen-antibody reaction
        D. When rabbit serum is used
        E. When agglutination of bacterial cells is observed

1453.   INFECTIOUS MONONUCLEOSIS IS CAUSED BY A(AN):
        A. Paramyxovirus
        B. Oncogenic virus
        C. Herpesvirus
        D. Bacteria
        E. Rickettsia

1454.   WHICH ONE OF THE FOLLOWING IS NOT A CHARACTERISTIC OF
        TYPHOID FEVER?
        A. Insidious onset, with malaise, anorexia, headache
        B. High polymorph leukocytosis and shift to the left
        C. Pulse slow compared to fever
        D. Rose spots
        E. Splenomegaly

1455. BETA HEMOLYTIC STREPTOCOCCI CAN BE DIFFERENTIATED
       FROM ALPHA AND GAMMA STRAINS ON BLOOD AGAR PLATES
       BY OBSERVING:
       A. Small colonies surrounded by a zone of hemolysis and a zone of
           discolored erythrocytes
       B. A clear zone of hemolysis
       C. No hemolysis
       D. Small colonies surrounded by a green ring
       E. A and B are correct

1456. URTICARIA IS USUALLY CAUSED BY:
       A. Noninfectious bacteria
       B. Allergy
       C. Virus
       D. Rickettsia
       E. Molds

1457. TO PRODUCE ACTIVE ARTIFICIAL IMMUNITY, THE PATIENT'S
       BODY:
       A. Is injected with sterile bacterial proteins
       B. Is injected with sterile bacterial antigens
       C. Is injected with living infectious organisms with attenuated virulence
       D. Is induced to produce antibodies against a specific disease
       E. All are correct

1458. A SCRATCH CAUSED BY RUSTY METAL MIGHT CAUSE:
       A. Typhoid fever
       B. Tetanus
       C. Undulant fever
       D. Murine typhus
       E. None of the above

1459. AGGLUTINATION REACTION IS USED FOR:
       A. Identifying bacteria
       B. Widal test
       C. Wassermann test
       D. A and C are correct
       E. A and B are correct

1460. THE POLIOMYELITIS VIRUS ORDINARILY ENTERS THE
       BODY THROUGH THE:
       A. Ear
       B. Skin
       C. Mouth
       D. Lungs
       E. None of the above

1461.   AN EXAMPLE OF IMMUNIZATION WITH ATTENUATED LIVING
        INFECTIOUS AGENT IS:
        A. Vaccination
        B. Anaphylaxis
        C. Any antigen injection
        D. Neisser-Wechsberg phenomenon
        E. Anabolism

1462.   THE U. S. P. H. S. IS A BRANCH OF:
        A. Department of Justice
        B. F. D. A.
        C. Dept. of HEW
        D. Dept. of Commerce
        E. FTC

1463.   IN THE U. S. MOST CASES OF BOTULISM CAN BE TRACED TO:
        A. Undercooked pork
        B. Home-canned sausage and other meats
        C. Home-canned vegetables and fruits
        D. Fish from polluted water
        E. Infected pastry

1464.   THE ORGANISM MOST COMMONLY FOUND IN THE INFECTIONS OF
        THE BONE IS:
        A. Meningococcus
        B. E. coli
        C. Staphylococcus pyogenes
        D. Mycobacterium tuberculosis
        E. Pseudomonas aeruginosa

1465.   VACCINE PREPARED FROM A PATIENT'S OWN INFECTION IS CALLED:
        A. Autogenous vaccine   D. Polyvalent vaccine
        B. Stock vaccine   E. Simple vaccine
        C. Monovalent vaccine

1466.   THE SUBSTANCE IN AIRPLANE GLUE MOST RESPONSIBLE FOR
        ADVERSE EFFECTS IS:
        A. Phenol
        B. Organic solvents
        C. Gums
        D. Alcohol
        E. Volatile oils

1467.   WATER IS UNFIT FOR HUMAN CONSUMPTION WHEN COLIFORM
        ORGANISMS ARE PRESENT BECAUSE:
        A. It contains bacteria
        B. It shows fecal contamination
        C. It indicates possible contamination by entering pathogens
        D. B and C are both correct
        E. None of the above

1468.   ACUTE LOBAR PNEUMONIA IS USUALLY CAUSED BY A(AN):
        A. Virus
        B. Bacteria
        C. Rickettsia
        D. All of the above
        E. None of the above

1469.   WHICH OF THE FOLLOWING ANTIBIOTICS IS USUALLY GIVEN
        ONLY ONCE DAILY FOR MAINTENANCE?
        A. Declomycin
        B. Vibramycin
        C. Achromycin
        D. Aureomycin
        E. Chloromycetin

1470.   WHICH OF THE FOLLOWING DISEASES IS NOT COMMONLY
        CONTRACTED THROUGH CONTAMINATED FOOD?
        A. Botulism
        B. Septic sore throat
        C. Typhoid
        D. Pyorrhea
        E. A and D are correct

FOR EACH OF THE FOLLOWING MULTIPLE CHOICE QUESTIONS
SELECT THE ONE MOST APPROPRIATE ANSWER:

1471.   _____ CONTAINS AN ETHYLENEDIAMINE NUCLEUS.
A. Chlortetracycline
B. Tripelennamine
C. Lidocaine
D. Pentobarbital
E. Pyrvinium pamoate

1472.   ALDEHYDES TEND TO PRODUCE _____ UPON OXIDATION.
A. Ketones   D. Acids
B. Alkanes   E. Ethers
C. Esters

1473.   WHICH OF THE FOLLOWING IS USED TO TEST FOR REDUCING SUGARS
IN URINE?
A. Acetest   D. Iodine
B. Benzidine reagent   E. None of these
C. Benedict's reagent

1474.   DUQUENOIS REAGENT WHEN ACIDIFIED PRODUCES A BLUE COLOR
IN THE PRESENCE OF:
A. Amphetamines   D. Marihuana
B. Barbiturates   E. STP
C. LSD

1475.   EDTA IS:
A. A monobasic acid   D. An ester
B. A polybasic acid   E. None of these
C. An imide

1476.   A CHROMOPHORE GROUP:
A. Intensifies a color
B. Weakens a color
C. Causes color
D. Has nothing to do with color
E. Is colored

1477.   MARQUIS REAGENT IN THE PRESENCE OF OPIUM ALKALOIDS GIVES
A _____ COLOR.
A. Red   D. Green
B. Orange   E. Yellow
C. Purple

1478.   STRYCHNINE PRODUCES A _____ COLOR IN THE PRESENCE
OF SULFURIC ACID AND POTASSIUM DICHROMATE.
A. Reddish-orange
B. Black
C. Yellow green
D. Blue-violet
E. Brown

1479.   IN THE ASSAY OF ACETIC ACID EACH CC OF 1N NaOH IS
        EQUIVALENT TO:
        A. 0.600 gm of acetic acid
        B. 0.00605 gm of acetic acid
        C. 0.06005 gm of acetic acid
        D. 6.005 gm of acetic acid
        E. 6.006 gm of acetic acid

1480.   ADDITION OF A FERRIC SALT TO A NEUTRAL SOLUTION OF AN
        ACETATE PRODUCES A DEEP _____ COLOR.
        A. Red   D. Blue
        B. Yellow   E. None of these
        C. Violet

1481.   TRICHLOROMETHANE IS ALSO CALLED:
        A. Methyl chloride   D. Freon
        B. Carbon tetrachloride   E. Chlorox
        C. Chloroform

1482.   CHLORAL HYDRATE IS USUALLY CLASSIFIED AS A(AN):
        A. Acid   D. Aldehyde
        B. Anydride   E. Ester
        C. Ketone

1483.   WHICH OF THE FOLLOWING INSTRUMENTS IS USED TO
        MEASURE SODIUM AND POTASSIUM IONS QUANTITATIVELY?
        A. Ion chamber
        B. Flame photometer
        C. Polarimeter
        D. Spectrophotometer
        E. Friabilator

1484.   THE PRINCIPAL HYDROLYSIS DEGRADATION PRODUCT OF
        ASPIRIN IS:
        A. Salicylic acid   D. Acrolein
        B. Methyl salicylate   E. Acetyl chloride
        C. Salicylamide

1485.   GRIGNARD REAGENTS USUALLY CONTAIN:
        A. Co   D. Pb
        B. Cu   E. Mg
        C. Fe

1486.   NMR IS USED MAINLY FOR:
        A. Assays
        B. Irradiation
        C. Identification of chemical substances
        D. Radioisotopes
        E. None of the above

1487.   CHEMICALLY, TETRACYCLINES ARE:
        A. Acids
        B. Bases
        C. Amphoteric
        D. Non-salt formers
        E. All esters

1488.   THE STEROID IDENTIFICATION TEST IN THE U. S. P. IS PRIMARILY
A (AN) _____ METHOD.
A. Chromatographic
B. Spectrophotometric
C. Acid-base titration
D. Gravimetric
E. Fluoroscopic

1489.   WHEN ASPIRIN IS HEATED WITH WATER FOR SEVERAL MINUTES,
COOLED, AND A DROP OR TWO OF FERRIC CHLORIDE T.S   IS
ADDED, A _____ COLOR DEVELOPS.
A. Blue   D. Green
B. Red   E. None of these
C. Violet

1490.   pH IS USUALLY MEASURED WITH:
A. A platinum electrode   D. A glass electrode
B. A mercury electrode   E. None of these
C. A copper electrode

1491.   THE PRINCIPLE OF THE REFRACTOMETRIC METHOD OF ANALYSIS
DEPENDS UPON:
A. Densities between two substances
B. Molecular weights of substances assayed
C. Volumes of substances assayed
D. Ultraviolet spectrum of substance being assayed
E. None of these

1492.   IODOMETRY IS:
A. A gravimetric method for the determination of iodine
B. Process of determining iodine volumetrically
C. Is an analytical method for the determination of iodides
D. None of these
E. All of these

1493.   MERCURY COMPOUNDS EXERT THEIR TOXIC EFFECTS BY TYING
UP:
A. Sulfhydryl groups   D. Carboxyl groups
B. Ester linkages   E. Double bonds
C. Lactones

1494.   THE VISIBLE RANGE OF LIGHT HAS A WAVE LENGTH RANGE OF:
A. 1000 to 6000 angstroms
B. 4000 to 7000 angstroms
C. 40-70 millimicrons
D. 10-60 millimicrons
E. 700-1100 angstroms

1495.   HOW MANY MOLECULES OF NaOH WILL REACT WITH 6.06×10^{23}
        MOLECULES OF SULFURIC ACID?
        A. 6.06×10^{23}
        B. 12.12×10^{23}
        C. 3.03×10^{23}
        D. 6.06×10^{46}
        E. $6.06 \times 10^{11.5}$

1496.   PARALDEHYDE IS FORMED BY POLYMERIZATION OF:
        A. Acetaldehyde
        B. Formaldehyde
        C. Propionaldehyde
        D. Ethanol
        E. Acetone

1497.   AN 18 CARBON ATOM SATURATED FATTY ACID IS:
        A. Myristic acid
        B. Lauric acid
        C. Oleic acid
        D. Stearic acid
        E. None of the above

MATCH THE FOLLOWING IONS WITH THE RESPECTIVE TESTS WHICH
ARE SPECIFIC FOR THEM (UNDER CERTAIN CONDITIONS):

1498. ___ Silver   A. Diphenyl-thiocarbazone
1499. ___ Lead   B. Quinoline-potassium iodide
1500. ___ Mercury (ous)   C. Diphenyl carbazide
1501. ___ Mercury (ic)   D. Dimethyl-aminobenzylidine rhodanine
1502. ___ Bismuth   E. Gallic acid

1503.   SUCROSE HYDROLIZES TO:
        A. Glucose
        B. Glucose and mannose
        C. Glucose and galactose
        D. Glucose and fructose
        E. Glucose and lactose

1504.   _____ CONTAINS SIXTEEN CARBON ATOMS.
        A. Arachidic acid
        B. Oleic acid
        C. Stearic acid
        D. Aspirin
        E. None of the above

MATCH THE FOLLOWING IONS WITH THE CHARACTERISTIC COLOR
GIVEN IN THE FLAME TEST:

1505. ___ Calcium   A. Green
1506. ___ Barium   B. Blue
1507. ___ Lead   C. Brick red
1508. ___ Potassium   D. Violet
1509. ___ Sodium   E. Yellow

128   SECTION IV - CHEMISTRY

MATCH THE FOLLOWING CHEMICAL NAMES WITH THE
CORRECT COMMON NAME:

1510. ___ Hydroxybenzene   A. Ether U.S.P.
1511. ___ Trichloromethane   B. Glycerin
1512. ___ Diethyl oxide   C. Toluene
1513. ___ Symmetrical trihydroxy propane   D. Chloroform
1514. ___ Methyl benzene   E. Phenol

1515.   TO AN UNKNOWN SOLUTION IS ADDED HCL AND H_2S WHICH
         YIELDS A BLACK PRECIPITATE. THE PRECIPITATE IS
         INSOLUBLE IN DILUTE YELLOW AMMONIUM SULFIDE BUT IS
         SOLUBLE IN NITRIC ACID. THE ION PRESENT IS:
         A. Bismuth
         B. Copper (ic)
         C. Mercury (ic)
         D. Ferrous
         E. Lead

1516.   AN UNKNOWN SOLUTION IS TREATED WITH HCL AND H_2S TO
         YIELD A BROWN PRECIPITATE WHICH DOES NOT DISSOLVE
         IN DILUTE YELLOW AMMONIUM SULFIDE SOLUTION. THE
         ION PRESENT IS:
         A. Lead
         B. Copper
         C. Silver
         D. Bismuth
         E. None of the above

1517.   WHICH OF THE FOLLOWING SALTS WOULD BE ACID IN REACTION
         WHEN DISSOLVED?
         A. Sodium lactate   D. Sodium chloride
         B. Magnesium carbonate   E. Potassium sulfate
         C. Antimony chloride

MATCH THE FOLLOWING:

1518. ___ Silver sulfide   A. Yellow
1519. ___ Silver iodide   B. White
1520. ___ Silver bromide   C. Black
1521. ___ Silver chloride   D. None of these

1522.   AN UNKNOWN SOLUTION IS TREATED WITH ACID PERMANGANATE
         AND THEN SHAKEN WITH CHLOROFORM. THE CHLOROFORM
         LAYER BECOMES COLORED BROWN TO AMBER. THE ION
         PRESENT IS:
         A. Silver
         B. Bromide
         C. Arsenate
         D. Copper
         E. Iodide

1523. TO AN UNKNOWN SOLUTION ACIDIFIED WITH ACETIC ACID IS
       ADDED POTASSIUM NITRITE. THE SOLUTION IS SHAKEN WITH
       CHLOROFORM. THE CHLOROFORM LAYER BECOMES VIOLET IN
       COLOR. THE ION PRESENT IS:
       A. Bromide   D. Silver
       B. Chloride   E. Ferricyanide
       C. Iodide

1524. AN UNKNOWN SOLUTION FORMS A CURDY WHITE PRECIPITATE
       UPON THE ADDITION OF HCL WHICH IS SOLUBLE IN EXCESS
       AMMONIUM HYDROXIDE. UPON ADDITION OF NITRIC ACID TO
       ACIDIFY THE SOLUTION, A WHITE PRECIPITATE FORMS. THE ION
       PRESENT IS:
       A. Silver   D. Bismuth
       B. Mercury (ous)   E. Calcium
       C. Lead

1525. A SOLUTION IS TREATED WITH HCL TO YIELD A WHITE PRECIPI-
       TATE WHICH IS INSOLUBLE IN HOT WATER OR EXCESS AMMONIUM
       HYDROXIDE. THE ION PRESENT IS:
       A. Lead   D. Cupric
       B. Silver   E. None of these
       C. Mercurous

1526. A SOLUTION IS TREATED WITH HCL AND H_2S TO YIELD A YELLOW
       PRECIPITATE WHICH IS INSOLUBLE IN AMMONIUM SULFIDE. THE
       ION PRESENT IS:
       A. Arsenic   D. Mercury
       B. Lead   E. Cadmium
       C. Bismuth

1527. A SOLUTION ACIDIFIED WITH HCL GIVES A YELLOW PRECIPITATE
       WITH H_2S WHICH IS SOLUBLE IN AMMONIUM SULFIDE AND INSO-
       LUBLE IN HCL. THE ION PRESENT IS:
       A. Tin   D. Copper
       B. Antimony   E. Arsenic
       C. Magnesium

1528. AN UNKNOWN SOLUTION FORMS A BROWN OR YELLOW PRECIPITATE
       IN AN ACID SOLUTION SATURATED WITH H_2S. THE PRECIPITATE IS
       SOLUBLE IN AMMONIUM POLYSULFIDE AND HCL. THE ION PRESENT
       IS:
       A. Arsenic
       B. Tin
       C. Antimony
       D. Lead
       E. Silver

MATCH THE FOLLOWING:

1529. ___ Pentobarbital   A. Amytal
1530. ___ Methohexital   B. Nembutal
1531. ___ Thiopental   C. Pentothal
1532. ___ Secobarbital   D. Brevital
1533. ___ Amobarbital   E. Seconal

1534. PHOSGENE GAS IS TOXIC BECAUSE:
       A. It relaxes free Cl_2
       B. It hydrolyzes to HCl
       C. It oxidizes to F_2
       D. It hydrolyzes to $CH Cl_3$
       E. None of the above

MATCH EACH DRUG OR CLASS OF DRUGS WITH AN AGENT
THAT WILL PRECIPITATE THEM:

1535. ___ Soluble barium salts   A. Carbon dioxide
1536. ___ Soluble silver salts   B. Halide ions
1537. ___ Alkaloids   C. Sulfates
1538. ___ Lime water   D. Nitric acid
1539. ___ Barbiturate salts   E. Mayer's reagent

1540. THE IONIZATION CONSTANT OF WATER AT 25° C IS:
       A. 7
       B. 14
       C. 1×10^{-7}
       D. 1×10^{7}
       E. 1×10^{-14}

1541. BARBITURATES CONTAINING A SULFUR ATOM ARE USUALLY:
       A. Ultra-short acting
       B. Unpredictable
       C. Short acting
       D. Intermediate acting
       E. Long acting

MATCH THE FOLLOWING IONS WITH THEIR RESPECTIVE
SPECIFIC TESTS:

1542. ___ Zinc   A. Flame test
1543. ___ Barium   B. Diphenylthiocarbazone
1544. ___ Strontium   C. 8-hydroxyquinoline
1545. ___ Calcium   D. Vapor-litmus paper test
1546. ___ Ammonium   E. None of these

MATCH THE FOLLOWING:

1547. ___ Boyle's Law
1548. ___ Avogadro's Law
1549. ___ Charles's Law

A. Equal volumes of gases under the same conditions of temperature
   and pressure contain the same number of molecules
B. The volume of a gas is inversely proportional to pressure if the
   temperature is constant
C. The pressure exerted by a gas is proportional to the absolute
   temperature if the volume of gas is kept constant

WHAT ARE THE PRODUCTS OF THE FOLLOWING REACTIONS ?

1550. ___ Phenols + acid anhydrides
1551. ___ NH_3 + a, b-unsaturated acids
1552. ___ Auto-oxidation of ethers
1553. ___ Aromatic hydrocarbons + acyl
          halides + anhydride alum. chloride
1554. ___ Aldehydes + alcohols + acid
          catalysts
1555. ___ Phenylhydrazine + aldehydes
1556. ___ Mercaptans + I_2 + NaOH
1557. ___ Zinc dust + disulfide + sulfuric acid
1558. ___ Acid halide + acid salt
1559. ___ Acyl halides + NH_3
1560. ___ Reduction of alkyl halide
1561. ___ Alcohols + inorganic acids

A. Peroxides
B. Oxazones
C. Mercaptans
D. Esters
E. Disulfides
F. Ketones
G. Acid anhydride
H. Amino acids
I. Amides
J. Acetals
K. Alkanes
L. Alkyl halides

1562. LE CHATELIER'S LAW OF MOBILE EQUILIBRIUM STATES THAT:
      " IF THE CONDITIONS OF A SYSTEM IN EQUILIBRIUM ARE
      ALTERED, ...
      A. Equilibrium cannot be reestablished"
      B. The equilibrium shifts in the direction which tends to neutralize
         the change in conditions"
      C. The equilibrium shifts in the direction which tends to accentuate the
         change in conditions"
      D. There is no change in the equilibrium"
      E. None of these

MATCH EACH SUBSTANCE WITH ITS pH IN AQUEOUS SOLUTION:

1563. ___ Sodium carbonate   A. Acid
1564. ___ Phenol
1565. ___ Potassium chloride   B. Alkaline
1566. ___ Sodium pentobarbital
                                      C. Neutral

1567. WHICH STATEMENT IS TRUE REGARDING:

$$Ag^+ + Cl^- \quad AgCl$$

A. If the ions corresponding to the "insoluble" substance are present in
    sufficient concentration to make their product greater than the
    solubility product then the solution is less than saturated
B. An "insoluble" salt will dissolve in a solution in which, for any
    reason, the product of the concentrations of its ions is less than the
    value of the solubility product
C. When ion product exceeds solution product no precipitate can occur
D. All of these
E. None of these

MATCH EACH SUBSTANCE WITH ITS PRIMARY CLASSIFICATION:

1568. ___ Aspirin   A. Barbiturate
1569. ___ Thioamylal   B. Aldehyde
1570. ___ Polysorbate 80   C. Ester
1571. ___ Chloral hydrate   D. Non-ionic surfactant

MATCH THE FOLLOWING:

1572. ___ Acid   A. Conjugate base of HCl
                                      B. Ionic or molecular sub-
1573. ___ Base   stance capable of giving up
                                          a proton to another sub-
1574. ___ Cl$^-$ stance
                                      C. Conjugate base of NH_4^+
1575. ___ NH$_3$ D. 1 gram molecular weight of
                                          reagent dissolved in 1000
1576. ___ Molal solution   gm. of solvent
                                      E. Proton acceptor

MATCH EACH GROUP OR TYPE OF DRUGS WITH THE CATION OR
ANION WITH WHICH IT IS MOST CLOSELY ASSOCIATED:

A. Mg

B. Organic nitrates

C. Cobalt

D. Potassium

E. Gold

F. Iron

1577. ___ Hematinics
1578. ___ Anti-arthritics
1579. ___ Treatment of muscle weakness
1580. ___ Treatment of angina
1581. ___ Antineoplastics
1582. ___ Antacids

1583. WHICH IS NOT TRUE OF SALTS?
       A. High melting points
       B. Soluble in water
       C. Solutions and melts are nonconducting
       D. Nonvolatile
       E. Insoluble in nonaqueous liquids

MATCH THE FOLLOWING:

A. Electrochemical equivalent of an element or group of elements
B. Amount of electricity required to liberate 1 gram equivalent weight
   of any substance
C. Milligrams of KOH required to neutralize free acids in 1 gm of a fat
D. Milligrams of KOH required to neutralize free and combined acids
   in 1 gm of fat
E. Number of mg of KOH required to saponify the esters in 1 gm of fat

1584. ___ Faraday
1585. ___ Acid value
1586. ___ Saponification value
1587. ___ Ester number
1588. ___ Coulomb

MATCH EACH OF THE FOLLOWING SUBSTANCES WITH ITS
CHEMICAL CLASSIFICATION:

1589. ___ Chloral hydrate   A. Ketone
1590. ___ Glycerin   B. Polyhydric alcohol
1591. ___ Acetone   C. Aldehyde

134   SECTION IV - CHEMISTRY

MATCH THE FOLLOWING:

A. Diazonium salts
B. Amides
C. Oxidation of mercaptans
D. Dehydrogenation of sec. alcohols
E. Ethers

1592. ___ Sulfonic acids can be prepared by ...
1593. ___ Heating ammonium carboxylates yields ...
1594. ___ The reaction of a metal alkoxide with an alkyl halide yields ...
1595. ___ Ketones may be prepared by ...
1596. ___ The actions of nitrous acid on the salt of an aromatic amine yields ...

A. Ratio of absolute viscosity in poises to the density
B. Based upon reflection of light
C. Force of friction that tends to retard movement in a fluid body
D. Based upon absorption of light

1597. ___ Viscosity
1598. ___ Nephelometry
1599. ___ Colorimetry
1600. ___ Kinematic viscosity

1601. ADSORPTION IS A(AN):
A. Irreversible chemical reaction
B. Reversible chemical reaction
C. Complexation phenomenon
D. Light-induced reaction
E. Physical phenomenon

MATCH EACH OF THE FOLLOWING SUBSTANCES TO THE
CLASSIFICATION IT FITS BEST: ·

1602. ___ Glycerin   A. Ester
1603. ___ Propylene glycol   B. Ketone
1604. ___ Aspirin   C. Polyhydric alcohol
1605. ___ Camphor   D. Amide
1606. ___ LSD   E. Alkaloid
1607. ___ Nicotine   F. Steroid
1608. ___ Ephedrine   G. Quinoline

1609. LONDON FORCES IN MOLECULES ARE:
A. Coordinate covalent bonds
B. Weak intramolecular forces
C. Strong intermolecular forces
D. Weak intermolecular forces
E. Hydrogen bonds

MATCH THE FOLLOWING:

1610. ___	Leuco base	A. d-1-amphetamine
1611. ___	Freezing point	B. 2 or more compounds with same
1612. ___	Isomers	molecular formula but differing in at
1613. ___	Racemic mixture	least one chemical or physical pro-
1614. ___	Mutarotation	perty
1615. ___	Van der Waals force	C. Used to calculate molecular weights
1616. ___	Enantiomorphs	D. Colorless form of a dye
		E. Change in optical rotation of a solu-
		tion of an optically active compound
		F. Increased attraction between mole-
		cules as the number of atoms
		increases
		G. 2 isomers that rotate plane polarized
		light equal amounts in opposite
		direction

MATCH THE FOLLOWING:

1617. ___	Methane	A. Alkyne
1618. ___	1-butene	B. Ester
1619. ___	Amyl nitrite	C. Mercaptan
1620. ___	Alkyl magnesium chloride	D. Polyhydric alcohol
1621. ___	Acetylene	E. Alkane
1622. ___	H_2NNH_2	F. Hydrazine
1623. ___	RSH	G. Aldose
1624. ___	Glucose	H. Alkene
1625. ___	Glycogen	I. Grignard reagent
1626. ___	Glycerin	J. Polysaccharide

1627. WHICH OF THE FOLLOWING HAS SPERMATOCIDAL ACTIVITY?
A. Lactic acid
B. Penicillinic acid
C. 17 Nor compounds
D. Oleic acid
E. Sodium phosphate

1628. WHICH IS USUALLY THE QUICKEST METHOD OF ANALYSIS?
A. Paper chromatography
B. TLC
C. Gas chromatography
D. Column chromatography
E. Spectrophotometry

1629. FLUORINATED HYDROCARBONS ARE OFTEN USED AS:
A. General anesthetics
B. Hypnotics
C. Anti-arrhythmics
D. Antihypertensives
E. Diuretics

1630.   WHAT IS THE MOST COMMONLY USED QUANTITATIVE METHOD
        FOR THE DETERMINATION OF NITROGEN IN ORGANIC COMPOUNDS?
        A.   Dumas
        B.   Nitrometer
        C.   Parr
        D.   Kjeldahl
        E.   Fiske-Subbarow

1631.   A REAGENT USED TO TEST FOR INDOLE STRUCTURES IS:
        A.   Dimethyl ketone
        B.   Formic acid
        C.   p-aminobenzaldehyde
        D.   Acetaldehyde
        E.   Benzoic acid

1632.   THE RATE OF ZERO ORDER REACTIONS:
        A.   Changes constantly
        B.   Is independent of temperature
        C.   Is independent of concentration
        D.   Holds only for light-catalyzed reactions
        E.   Holds only for radioactive compounds

1633.   A NORMAL SOLUTION CONTAINS:
        A.   1 gm equivalent weight of solute in 1000 gm of solution
        B.   1 gm equivalent weight of solute in 1000 cc of solvent
        C.   1 gm equivalent weight of solute in 1000 cc of solution
        D.   1 gm molecular weight of solute in 1000 cc of solvent
        E.   1 gm molecular weight of solute in 1000 cc of solution

1634.   A FIXED OIL IS:
        A.   Glyceryl esters of saturated fatty acids
        B.   Glyceryl esters of unsaturated fatty acids
        C.   Glyceryl esters of saturated and unsaturated fatty acids
        D.   Any ester of fatty acids
        E.   Any ester of unsaturated fatty acids

1635.   WHICH OF THE FOLLOWING SUBSTANCES IS ENDOTHERMIC
        WHEN DISSOLVED?
        A.   Sodium hydroxide
        B.   Sulfuric acid
        C.   Potassium iodide
        D.   Nitric acid
        E.   None of the above

1636.   DETERMINATION OF IODINE VALUE DEPENDS UPON:
        A.   Substitution with iodine for the hydrogen in the fatty acids
        B.   Addition of iodine at the double bond of fatty acids
        C.   Oxidation of the fatty acids by iodine
        D.   Analysis of the iodine content of a fatty acid
        E.   None of the above

1637.   MOST OF THE LOCAL ANESTHETICS ARE:
A. Esters of salicylic acid
B. Esters of p-aminobenzoic acid
C. Amides of naphthoic acid
D. Esters of propionic acid
E. Allantoin derivatives

1638.   THE pH OF SOLUTIONS OF SODIUM BORATE TEND TO BE:
A. Strongly acidic
B. Weakly acidic
C. Neutral
D. Weakly alkaline
E. Strongly alkaline

1639.   WHICH OF THE FOLLOWING COULD BE USED AS A REDUCING
AGENT?
A. Potassium permanganate
B. Glucose
C. Potassium dichromate
D. Barium sulfate
E. None

1640.   AMPHETAMINE IS:
A. Phenylethanolamine
B. Desoxyephedrine
C. Desoxynorephedrine
D. Desoxynorepinephrine
E. None of the above

1641.   TANNINS ARE VERY INCOMPATIBLE WITH:
A. All acids
B. All ionic salts
C. All ferric salts
D. All glycosides
E. All potassium salts

1642.   DEUTERIUM IS A RADIOACTIVE FORM OF WHICH ELEMENT?
A. Carbon
B. Oxygen
C. Hydrogen
D. Iodine
E. Cobalt

1643.   A SACCHARIMETER MEASURES:
A. Light transmittance
B. Optical rotation
C. Light absorption
D. Refractive index
E. None of the above

1644.   ARGYROL IS A(AN):
        A. Colloidal silver compound
        B. Mercury compound
        C. Sulfite
        D. Completely inorganic compound
        E. Nonionizable compound

1645.   WHICH OF THE FOLLOWING CHEMICALS IS CONSIDERED TO BE
        VERY WATER SOLUBLE?
        A. Mercuric chloride
        B. Mercurous chloride
        C. Silver chloride
        D. Barium sulfate
        E. Calcium sulfate

FOR EACH OF THE FOLLOWING MULTIPLE CHOICE QUESTIONS
SELECT THE ONE MOST APPROPRIATE ANSWER:

1646.   THE SULFUR-CONTAINING AMINO ACID IS:
         A. Valine   D. Glutamic acid
         B. Glycine   E. Histidine
         C. Cystine

1647.   METHIONINE IS A (AN):
         A. Narcotic analgesic   D. Vitamin
         B. Essential amino acid   E. Coenzyme
         C. Hormone

MATCH EACH DIAGNOSTIC TO THE FUNCTION IT IS USED TO DETECT:

1648. ___ Histamine phosphate   A. Kidney function
1649. ___ Betazole HCl   B. Gastric acid secretion
1650. ___ Phenol red   C. Liver function

1651.   WHICH AMINO ACID IS RELATED TO THYROXINE:
         A. Tyrosine   D. Threonine
         B. Tyramine   E. Cysteine
         C. Tryptophane

1652.   WHICH IS NOT AN ESSENTIAL AMINO ACID?
         A. Threonine   D. Glutamine
         B. Tryptophane   E. Methionine
         C. Valine

1653.   INSULIN IS USUALLY CLASSIFIED AS:
         A. A protein
         B. An amino acid
         C. A phospholipid
         D. An enzyme
         E. A hormone

1654.   AN ENZYME IS A SUBSTANCE WHICH:
         A. Hydrolyzes
         B. Dehydrates
         C. Converts heat to energy
         D. Acts as a catalyst
         E. Is changed chemically in a reaction

1655.   A SUBSTANCE FOUND COMMONLY IN FERMENTED FOODS WHICH CAN
         BE TOXIC WHEN MAO INHIBITORS ARE USED IS:
         A. ADP   D. Histidine
         B. STP   E. Phenylalanine
         C. Tyramine

1656.   MAN IS MOST SENSITIVE TO THE _____ TASTE.
         A. Sour
         B. Sweet
         C. Bitter
         D. Salty
         E. Alkaline

1657. WHICH OF THE FOLLOWING IS NEEDED IN DETERMINING THE
ISOELECTRIC POINT OF AN AMINO ACID?
A. Structural formula
B. Dissociation constant
C. Electrophoretic pattern
D. Composition
E. pH

1658. THE CONVERSION OF AN AMINO ACID TO A SUGAR IS:
A. Hydrolysis   D. Glucogenesis
B. Cocarboxylation   E. None of these
C. Glycolysis

1659. BIOTIN IS ALSO SOMETIMES CALLED:
A. Vitamin B-6   D. Vitamin B-4
B. Vitamin H   E. Tocopherol
C. Vitamin B-12

1660. MAO IS CLASSIFIED AS:
A. A protein inhibitor
B. A complexing agent
C. An enzyme
D. A hormone
E. An amino acid

1661. WHICH OF THE FOLLOWING SUBSTANCES COULD BE RESPONSIBLE
FOR AN ELEVATION OF BLOOD PRESSURE?
A. Acetone bodies   D. Oxalic acid
B. Uric acid   E. Allantoin
C. Renin

1662. WHICH SUBSTANCE YIELDS THE LARGEST NUMBER OF CALORIES
PER GRAM?
A. Carbohydrates   D. Fats
B. Proteins   E. Vitamins
C. Minerals

1663. THE LETHAL EFFECT OF CO IS DUE TO ITS:
A. Vapor pressure
B. H_2O solubility
C. Ability to form CO_2 easily
D. Ability to combine with hemoglobin
E. Ability for forming a stable complex with myoglobin

1664. WHICH IONS ARE INVOLVED IN UPTAKE OF RENAL STONES?
A. Iron and cobalt
B. Sodium and potassium
C. Calcium and sodium
D. Chloride and bicarbonate
E. Chloride and oxalate

1665. INVERT SUGAR IS:
A. Maltose
B. Sucrose
C. Glucose
D. Levulose
E. Galactose

1666. WHICH OF THE FOLLOWING DRUGS IS LEAST LIKELY TO CAUSE ELECTROLYTE IMBALANCE?
A. Chlorothiazide
B. Aluminum hydroxide
C. Potassium chloride
D. Ethacrynic acid
E. Sodium bicarbonate

1667. NINHYDRIN IS A REAGENT USED EXTENSIVELY TO DETERMINE:
A. CO_2
B. Glucose
C. Hemoglobin
D. Amino acids
E. None of the above

1668. THE COENZYMES OF THE DEHYDROGENASES INCLUDE ALL OF THE FOLLOWING, EXCEPT:
A. DPN
B. Coenzyme II
C. FAD
D. Apoenzyme
E. FMN (Flavin Adenine Mononucleotide)

1669. DEFICIENCY OF FOLIC ACID WILL CAUSE:
A. Anemia
B. Rickets
C. Night blindness
D. Beri-beri
E. Diabetes

1670. A COMPONENT OF COENZYME A IS:
A. Inosine
B. Thiamine
C. Pantothenic acid
D. Triphosphopyridine nucleotide
E. Acetate

1671. A NORMAL VALUE FOR NPN IN BLOOD IS:
A. 0 mg %
B. 5-10 mg %
C. 10-20 mg %
D. 25-40 mg %
E. 100-150 mg %

1672. EPINEPHRINE AND NOREPINEPHRINE ARE SYNTHESIZED FROM:
A. Glycine
B. Argenine
C. Phenol
D. Catechol
E. Tyrosine

1673. THE MAJOR BUFFER OF THE EXTRACELLULAR FLUID IS:
A. Bicarbonate-CO_2 system
B. Phosphate
C. Protein
D. Sodium
E. None of these

1674. AN EXCESS OF NITROGENOUS WASTE IN THE BLOOD CAUSES:
A. Acidosis
B. Alkalosis
C. Kidney stones
D. Uremia
E. None of these

1675. THE NORMAL BLOOD CHEMISTRY VALUE OF SODIUM IN SERUM IN MG % IS:
A. 310-340
B. 50-100
C. 18-20
D. 390-450
E. 25-40

1676. THE SYNTHESIS OF NEW PROTEIN IN GROWTH TISSUE GENERALLY DEPENDS ON:
A. Carbohydrates
B. Fats
C. Iodine
D. Copper
E. Amino acids

1677. WHICH MAY GIVE A FALSE + IN THE 5-HIAA TESTS FOR CARCINOMA?
A. NaCl
B. Glyceryl guaiacolate
C. KCl
D. Tetracycline
E. Ampicillin

1678. THE ACTIVE PROTEOLYTIC ENZYME IN GASTRIC JUICE IS:
A. Pepsinogen
B. Pepsin
C. Bilirubin
D. Trypsin
E. Secretin

1679. A NEGATIVE NITROGEN BALANCE COULD OCCUR:
A. During normal pregnancy
B. In malnutrition
C. During normal child growth
D. During convalescence
E. None of the above

1680. HYPERVENTILATION CAUSES PROBLEMS BECAUSE IT TENDS TO DEPLETE:
A. Oxygen
B. Air
C. CO_2
D. Nitrogen
E. None of these

1681. _____ ENHANCES ACTIVITY OF AZATHIOPRINE BY INHIBITING ENZYMATIC OXIDATION?
A. Allopurinol
B. Elase
C. Dipyridamole
D. Trimethoprim
E. Tranylcypromine

1682.   ONE OF THE FOLLOWING IS NOT AN ENZYME INVOLVED IN
        GLYCOLYSIS:
        A. Enolase   D. Pyruvate kinase
        B. Diaphorase   E. Hexokinase
        C. Glycerophosphate dehydrogenase

1683.   THE END PRODUCT OF THE HYDROLYSIS OF GLYCOGEN IS:
        A. Galactose   D. Xylose
        B. Mannose   E. Arabinose
        C. Glucose

1684.   PORPHYRINS ARE INVOLVED IN THE BUILDING OF:
        A. Bones   D. Blood
        B. Teeth   E. Scar tissue
        C. Muscle

1685.   CERTAIN SUBSTANCES WHEN INJECTED ALONE DO NOT GIVE RISE
        TO THE FORMATION OF ANTIBODIES; THESE ARE DESIGNATED AS:
        A. Proteins   D. Haptens
        B. Exotoxins   E. Toxins
        C. Antitoxins

1686.   A NORMAL VALUE FOR GLUCOSE IN BLOOD IS:
        A. 250-350 mg. %   D. 80-120 mg. %
        B. 200-250 mg. %   E. 50-75 mg. %
        C. 100-200 mg. %

1687.   WHICH WILL DISPLACE COUMARIN FROM BINDING SITES?
        A. Insulin   D. Tolbutamide
        B. Norepinephrine   E. Ephedrine
        C. Acetylcholine

1688.   BETWEEN THE PARTICULATE AND MICELLAR CONSTITUENTS OF
        CELLS THERE EXISTS AN AQUEOUS PHASE WHICH CONTAINS:
        A. Soluble proteins
        B. Organic substances such as glucose
        C. Cellular active products such as creatine
        D. Electrolytes
        E. All of these

1689.   WHICH MAY GIVE A FALSE + GLUCOSE WITH TES-TAPE?
        A. Vitamin B_1 D. Erythromycin
        B. Vitamin E   E. Vitamin C
        C. Tetracycline

1690.   WHICH OF THE FOLLOWING IS CLASSIFIED AS A POLYSACCHARIDE?
        A. Saccharin
        B. Starch
        C. Lactose
        D. Sodium cyclamine
        E. Maltose

1691.   IN THE TYPICAL CELL, THE MITOCHONDRIA CONTAINS:
        A. Cytochrome oxidase
        B. Succinic acid oxidase
        C. Cytochrome C
        D. All of the above
        E. None of the above

1692.   THE MAIN CARBOHYDRATE OF THE BLOOD IS:
        A. D-fructose   D. Sorbitose
        B. Mannitol   E. L-glucose
        C. D-glucose

1693.   THE PRESENCE OF MITOCHONDRIA IN LIVING CELLS CAN BE
        DETERMINED BY THE USE OF:
        A. Neutral red   D. Phenolphthalein
        B. Methylene blue   E. None of these
        C. Janus green

1694.   _____ IS SOMETIMES CLASSIFIED AS A VITAMIN.
        A. Choline   D. Fructose
        B. DNA   E. Manganese
        C. RNA

1695.   WHICH DRUG IS LIKELY TO ELEVATE THE VALUE IN THE PBI TEST?
        A. Lithium carbonate   D. Aspirin
        B. INH   E. Potassium iodide
        C. Disulfiram

1696.   THE ENZYME IN SALIVA WHICH ACTS ON STARCH AND GLYCOGEN:
        A. Pepsinogen   D. Ptyalin
        B. Pepsin   E. Salivary calculus
        C. Rennin

1697.   BACTERIA WHICH REQUIRE PARA-AMINOBENZOIC ACID FOR
        THEIR GROWTH CAN BE INHIBITED BY:
        A. Folic acid   D. Adenine
        B. Folinic acid   E. Phenylalanine
        C. Sulfonamides

1698.   PRECURSOR OF THE ENZYME PEPSIN FORMED IN ALKALINE
        SOLUTION IS:
        A. Mucin
        B. Pepsinogen
        C. Ptyalin
        D. Rennin
        E. Lipase

1699.   A DEFICIENCY OF VITAMIN _____ CAN CAUSE NIGHT BLINDNESS.
        A. D
        B. K
        C. A
        D. E
        E. B complex

1700. _____ ACTS BY SPLITTING PROTEINS AT THE DISULFIDE
BOND.
A. Epinephrine   D. Oxytriphylline
B. INH   E. Phenylbutazone
C. N-acetylcysteine

1701. VITAMIN E IS ALSO KNOWN AS:
A. Niacin   D. Carotene
B. Tocopherol   E. Pteroylglutamic acid
C. Thiamine

1702. THE CONVERSION OF BETA-CAROTENE TO VITAMIN A IS
CARRIED OUT IN THE:
A. Liver   D. Thymus
B. Pancreas   E. Adrenal cortex
C. Spleen

1703. THE HEAT-LABILE FACTOR IN THE VITAMIN B COMPLEX IS:
A. Riboflavin   D. Folic acid
B. Biotin   E. Niacin
C. Thiamine

1704. BLOOD CLOTTING CAN BE PREVENTED BY:
A. Sodium chloride
B. Potassium chloride
C. Sodium citrate
D. Lithium chloride
E. All of the above

1705. WHICH IS MOST LIKELY TO ELEVATE THE VALUE OF A BUN TEST?
A. Tetracycline   D. Ampicillin
B. Penicillin G   E. Cromolyn sodium
C. Benzathine penicillin

1706. PANCREATIN IS USED THERAPEUTICALLY FOR:
A. Coughs
B. Pneumonia
C. Cystic fibrosis
D. Kidney failure
E. Cirrhosis

1707. WHICH OF THE FOLLOWING IS PRESENT IN ALL CONNECTIVE
TISSUE?
A. Mucoids   D. All of these
B. Lipids   E. None of these
C. Albuminoid

1708. PHYTONADIONE (VITAMIN K_1) IS USED TO TREAT:
A. Hematuria
B. Cystic fibrosis
C. Hemorrhagic disease of newborn
D. Agranulocytosis
E. Leukemias

1709.   IN THE ELECTROPHORETIC PROCESS AT A pH BELOW THE ISO-
        ELECTRIC POINT, A PROTEIN WILL:
        A.   Migrate to negative pole   D.   Form a Zwitter ion
        B.   Migrate to positive pole   E.   None of these
        C.   Exhibit no migration

1710.   THE CHIEF PIGMENT OF SKIN IS:
        A.   Eludin   D.   Glucose
        B.   Hyaline   E.   Melanin
        C.   Dihydroxyphenylalanine

1711.   KERATIN IS A (AN):
        A.   Protein   D.   Peptone
        B.   Albuminoid   E.   Histone
        C.   Glutelin

1712.   THE PELLAGRA PREVENTIVE FACTOR IN THE VITAMIN B COMPLEX:
        A.   Inositol
        B.   Pantothenic acid
        C.   Riboflavin
        D.   Niacin
        E.   Para-aminobenzoic acid

1713.   ALBUMINS AND GLOBULINS ARE CLASSIFIED AS:
        A.   Derived proteins   D.   Simple proteins
        B.   Waxes   E.   Enzymes
        C.   Conjugated proteins

1714.   VITAMIN K IS NECESSARY FOR:
        A.   Prevention of rickets   D.   Formation of DNA
        B.   Prevention of pernicious anemia   E.   Muscle tone
        C.   Formation of prothrombin

1715.   DEHYDROCHOLIC ACID IS USED TO TREAT:
        A.   Indigestion   D.   Ulcers
        B.   Diarrhea   E.   C and D
        C.   Gastritis

1716.   _____ FURNISHES MUCH ENERGY TO MUSCLES.
        A.   ACTH   D.   DNA
        B.   LSD   E.   ATP
        C.   RNA

1717.   ORAL CONTRACEPTIVES EXERT THEIR EFFECT PRIMARILY BY:
        A.   Preventing fertilization of the egg
        B.   Suppressing ovulation
        C.   Inactivating sperm
        D.   Preventing menses
        E.   None of the above

MATCH EACH SUBSTANCE WITH THE SITE OF SECRETION OR
FORMATION:

1718. ___ Pepsinogen   A. Pancreas
1719. ___ Bile salts   B. Zymogen cells
1720. ___ Insulin   C. Adrenal medulla
1721. ___ Norepinephrine   D. Liver

1722. WHICH OF THE FOLLOWING ARE ANTICOAGULANT AGENTS?
A. Fibrinolysin
B. Dicumarol
C. Hirudin
D. Heparin
E. All of these

1723. A COMBINATION OF L-DOPA AND _____ WILL CAUSE DE-
PLETION OF CATECHOLAMINES.
A. Carbidopa   D. Riboflavin
B. Amantadine   E. A and B
C. Chlorpromazine

1724. THE BENZIDINE TEST IS USED TO TEST FOR:
A. Uric acid   D. Blood
B. Alkaloids   E. Lipids
C. Amino acids

1725. THE ENZYME RESPONSIBLE FOR THE CONVERSION OF
GLYCOGEN TO GLUCOSE-1-PHOSPHATE IN MUSCLE TISSUE IS:
A. Aldolase
B. Phosphorylase
C. Carboxylase
D. Alcohol dehydrogenase
E. Enolase

1726. _____ PROTECTS THE BRAIN AND SPINAL CORD AGAINST
MECHANICAL INJURY.
A. The diencephalon   D. Acetylcholine
B. Norepinephrine   E. The blood-brain barrier
C. Cerebrospinal fluid

1727. THE FOLLICLE STIMULATING HORMONE (PROLACTIN) AND THE
INTERSTITIAL CELL-STIMULATING HORMONE ARE PRODUCED BY:
A. Islets of Langerhans
B. Thymus gland
C. Thyroid gland
D. Pineal gland
E. Pituitary gland

1728. _____ IS CAPABLE OF EITHER RELEASING DOPAMINE OR
DELAYING ITS DESTRUCTION.
A. Trihexyphenidyl
B. Benztropine
C. L-DOPA
D. Orphenadrine
E. Amantadine

1729.   REMOVAL OF WHICH GLANDS RESULTS IN LOW CALCIUM LEVEL
        IN BLOOD AND LEADS TO TETANY AND DEATH?
        A. Thyroid   D. Parathyroid
        B. Endocrine   E. None of these
        C. Adrenal

1730.   THE AVERAGE LIFE OF A RED BLOOD CELL IS ABOUT:
        A. 7 days   D. 1 to 2 months
        B. 14 days   E. 4 months
        C. 3 weeks

1731.   THE PRECURSORS OF VITAMIN A ARE:
        A. Proteins   D. Carotenes
        B. Tocopherols   E. Calciferols
        C. Erogosterols

1732.   THE VITAMIN WHICH PLAYS THE LARGEST PART IN THE PREVEN-
        TION OF DEGENERATIVE CHANGES IN THE CENTRAL NERVOUS
        SYSTEM IS:
        A. A   D. D
        B. B complex   E. K
        C. C

1733.   THE MAJOR CATEGORIES OF PROTEINS INTO WHICH NEARLY ALL
        ANTIBODIES FALL ARE:
        A. Gamma globulins   D. Leucosins
        B. Serum albumins   E. Glutelins
        C. Haptoglobins

1734.   THE USUAL SOURCE OF HEPARIN IS:
        A. Blood   D. From plants
        B. Fish   E. Synthetic
        C. Tissues of domestic mammals

1735.   THE PROTEIN PRECURSOR OF THYROXINE IS:
        A. Ornithine   D. Thyroglobulin
        B. Threonine   E. Thyroxinogen
        C. Tryptophane

1736.   A MILKY OR TURBID BLOOD PLASMA SAMPLE TAKEN 4-5 HOURS
        AFTER MEALS WOULD INDICATE INGESTION OF LARGE QUANTITIES
        OF:
        A. Vitamins
        B. Sugar
        C. Proteins
        D. Fats
        E. Minerals

1737.   IRON IN THE FORM OF FERRITIN IS STORED IN THE:
        A. Liver   D. Bone marrow
        B. Intestinal mucosa   E. All of these
        C. Spleen

MATCH THE ORGAN OR GLAND IN COLUMN II WITH THE
SUBSTANCE IT RELEASES IN COLUMN I:

COLUMN I   COLUMN II

1738. ___ Insulin   A. Thyroid
1739. ___ Pepsin   B. Liver
1740. ___ Thyroxin   C. Stomach
1741. ___ Arginase   D. Pancreas
1742. ___ Maltase   E. Small intestine

1743.   GIGANTISM AND ACROMEGALY ARE DISEASES ATTRIBUTED
        TO MALFUNCTION OF:
        A. Pineal gland   D. Pituitary gland
        B. Thymus gland   E. Gonads
        C. Islets of Langerhans

1744. CO_2 TRANSPORT IS EFFECTED THROUGH THE MEDIATION OF:
        A. DPN   D. Carbonic anhydrase
        B. TPN   E. Diamine oxidase
        C. Xanthine oxidase

1745.   MOST NITROGEN HETEROCYCLES ARE DETOXIFIED BY:
        A. Methylation
        B. Reduction
        C. Oxidation
        D. Hippuric acid
        E. Transconversion

1746.   THE pH OF BLOOD IS NORMALLY IN THE RANGE OF:
        A. 6.25 - 7.00
        B. 6.75 - 7.25
        C. 7.0 - 7.3
        D. 7.5 - 7.7
        E. 7.35 - 7.45

1747.   THE FEEDING OF VITAMIN B_{12} TO PERNICIOUS ANEMIA
        PATIENTS OVERCOMES:
        A. The lack of intrinsic factor
        B. The lack of extrinsic factor
        C. Lack of hydrochloric acid production
        D. Folic acid deficiency
        E. All of the above

1748.   APPROXIMATELY _____% OF THE POPULATION ARE Rh POSITIVE.
        A. 30%   D. 85%
        B. 50%   E. 95%
        C. 60%

1749.   THE FAT SOLUBLE VITAMINS ARE:
        A. B complex, C and D
        B. A, D, E, and K
        C. A, B, C, and D
        D. B complex, E, and K
        E. A, B complex, and D

1750.   LANDSTEINER'S CLASSIFICATION IS USED FOR:
        A. Blood typing
        B. Enzymes
        C. Proteins
        D. Carbohydrates
        E. Diabetics

1751.   TO AVOID PITUITARY HYPOFUNCTION _____ THERAPY
        SHOULD BE DISCONTINUED GRADUALLY.
        A. Diphenylhydantoin
        B. Potassium chloride
        C. ACTH
        D. Primidone
        E. Trimethadione

1752.   THE THERAPEUTIC ANTICONVULSANT LEVEL OF PHENOBARBITAL IS:
        A. 1-2 mcg/ml   D. 25-40 mcg/ml
        B. 2-10 mcg/ml   E. 50-60 mcg/ml
        C. 10-25 mcg/ml

1753.   THE ENZYME CARBONIC ANHYDRASE IS MARKEDLY INHIBITED BY:
        A. Salicylates
        B. Phenolic compounds
        C. Sulfonamides
        D. Fluorides
        E. Malonates

1754.   STARCHES ARE PARTIALLY DIGESTED IN THE MOUTH BY:
        A. Protease   D. Pepsin
        B. Pepsinogen   E. Ptyalin
        C. Rennin

1755.   THE HUMAN BODY STORES VITAMIN A IN:
        A. The liver
        B. The spleen
        C. The intestine
        D. Fat depots
        E. Muscle tissue

1756.   THE METABOLIC DEGRADATION OF HEMOGLOBIN TAKES PLACE
        PRINCIPALLY IN:
        A. The reticulo-endothelial system   D. The kidney tubules
        B. The RBC   E. All of these
        C. The liver cells

1757.   THE METABOLIC BREAKDOWN OF HEMOGLOBIN IN THE MAMMAL
        INVOLVES:
        A. The formation of bile pigments
        B. No oxidative cleavage of the porphyrin ring
        C. The formation of urobilin
        D. The formation of biliverdin
        E. All of these

MATCH THE USUAL NORMAL RANGE TO EACH OF THE
FOLLOWING LABORATORY TESTS:

1758. ___ RBC (men)		A. 4.5 to 6.5 million
1759. ___ WBC		B. 150-200 mg %
1760. ___ RBC (women)		C. 4000 to 11,000
1761. ___ Lymphocytes		D. 4 to 5.5 million
1762. ___ Serum NPN		E. 15 to 22 mg %
1763. ___ Serum potassium		F. 28-40 mg %
1764. ___ Serum cholesterol (total)		G. 1000 to 5000

1765. THE NONPROTEIN PORTION OF HEMOGLOBIN CONSISTS OF:
    A. 3 heme units surrounding an iron atom
    B. 4 heme units surrounding a ferric atom
    C. A ferrous complex of protoporphyrin IX
    D. 4 pyrrole rings linked through a ferric molecule
    E. None of the above

1766. THE FOLLOWING AMINO ACID IS AN IMPORTANT PRECURSOR
OF HEMOGLOBIN:
    A. Alanine   D. Leucine
    B. Proline   E. Histidine
    C. Glycine

1767. IN MOST MAMMALS, EXCEPT MAN AND THE HIGHER APES, URIC
ACID IS METABOLIZED BY:
    A. Reduction to ammonia
    B. Oxidation to allantoin
    C. Degradation to nitrogen
    D. Hydrolysis to ammonia
    E. Oxidation to ammonia and carbon dioxide

1768. IN MAN, THE PRINCIPAL END PRODUCT OF PURINE
METABOLISM IS:
    A. Nitrogen   D. Urea
    B. Ammonia   E. None of these
    C. Uric acid

1769. IN MAN, THE MAJOR NITROGENOUS EXCRETION PRODUCT IS:
    A. Amino acids
    B. Ammonia
    C. Nitrogen
    D. Purines and pyrimidines
    E. None of the above

1770. WHY IS QUINIDINE CONTRAINDICATED IN MYASTHENIA GRAVIS?
    A. Causes agranulocytosis
    B. Causes muscle spasm
    C. Causes ataxia
    D. Produces coma
    E. Inhibits neuromuscular transmission

1771.   WHICH VITAMIN IS USED OCCASIONALLY AS AN ANTIOXIDANT?
        A. Vitamin D   D. Vitamin E
        B. Vitamin K   E. Vitamin B_2
        C. Vitamin B_1

1772.   _____ IS RESPONSIBLE FOR THE TRANSFER OF
        GENETIC INFORMATION.
        A. ATP   D. STP
        B. RNA   E. None of these
        C. DNA

1773.   UREASE IS CLASSIFIED AS:
        A. An esterase   D. A peptidase
        B. An amidase   E. An oxidase
        C. A phosphorylase

1774.   A REACTION BETWEEN AN ANTIGEN AND AN ANTIBODY
        REQUIRES:
        A. Precipitin   D. High titer
        B. Complement factor   E. Low titer
        C. Heat above 50^0 C

1775.   PTYALIN IS A(N):
        A. Lipase   D. Amylase
        B. Anhydrase   E. Proteinase
        C. Urease

1776.   AEROBIC RESPIRATION IN CELLS IS MOSTLY CARRIED OUT IN THE:
        A. Mitochondria
        B. Nucleus
        C. Endoplasmic reticulum
        D. Cytoplasmic portion
        E. Microsomes

1777.   A TEST FOR CREATININE IN URINE IS:
        A. The Millon test
        B. The Schick test
        C. The Van Slyke test
        D. The Jaffe test
        E. The silver mirror test

1778.   AN IMPORTANT ENZYMATIC REACTION INVOLVED IN MUSCULAR
        CONTRACTION IS:
        A. Glucose-6-phosphatase reaction
        B. Glycogenolysis
        C. ATP-creatine transphosphorylase reaction
        D. Enolase reaction
        E. All of these

1779. BILE IS FORMED IN THE:
A. Stomach
B. Small intestine
C. Pancreas
D. Spleen
E. Liver

1780. BILE IS STORED IN THE:
A. Gallbladder
B. Spleen
C. Liver
D. Small intestine
E. Kidney

1781. THE ORAL HYPOGLYCEMIC AGENTS:
A. Inhibit release of liver glycogen
B. Have a direct insulin effect
C. Stimulate release of insulin from the pancreas
D. Act mainly by chemical reduction of glucose
E. None of the above

1782. DEATH DUE TO CYANIDE POISONING RESULTS FROM:
A. Cyanide-hemoglobin complex formation
B. Cyanide combining with the red blood cell
C. Cyanide inhibiting cytochrome oxidase
D. Coronary vessel occlusion
E. None of the above

1783. AN ENZYME COMMONLY FOUND IN SNAKE VENOM IS:
A. Urease
B. Ptyalin
C. Steapsin
D. Hyaluronidase
E. Catalase

1784. THE INACTIVE FORM OF AN ENZYME IS CALLED:
A. Kinase
B. Zymogen
C. Catalyst
D. Precursor enzyme
E. None of the above

1785. THE PHYSIOLOGICAL IMPORTANCE OF HEMOGLOBIN LIES
IN ITS ABILITY:
A. To combine irreversibly with oxygen and carbon dioxide
B. To combine reversibly with oxygen at the ferric portion of the
molecule
C. To combine irreversibly with oxygen at the ferrous portion of the
molecule
D. To combine reversibly with oxygen at the ferrous portion of the
molecule

1786. PEPSIN IS PRIMARILY A(AN):
A. Oxidase
B. Carbohydrase
C. Esterase
D. Peptidase
E. Protease

1787.   ACIDIC SUBSTANCES WILL _____ AMINOPHYLLINE.
      A. Not affect   D. Potentiate
      B. Precipitate   E. C and D
      C. Solubilize

1788.   THE VISUAL IMPULSE IS ASSOCIATED WITH THE:
      A. Photochemical transformation of rhodopsin
      B. The reduction of TPN
      C. The condensation of opsin with vitamin C
      D. The hydrolysis of visual purple
      E. All of the above

1789.   COENZYMES OFTEN CONTAIN A(AN) GROUP:
      A. Steroidal   D. Vitamin
      B. Protein   E. Amino acid
      C. Polypeptide

1790.   THE BIOCHEMICAL ROLE OF THE CAROTENOIDS LIES IN
      THEIR CONVERSION TO:
      A. Folic acid   D. Vitamin A
      B. Folinic acid   E. None of these
      C. Ascorbic acid

1791.   THE BIOLOGICAL HALF LIFE OF PHENYTOIN H IS:
      A. 1-2 hours
      B. 4-8 hours
      C. 14-16 hours
      D. 18-24 hours
      E. Over 24 hours

1792.   _____ STIMULATES HEPATIC MICROSOMAL ENZYMES.
      A. Phenacemide   D. Urea
      B. Mannitol   E. ASA
      C. Phenobarbital

1793.   VITAMIN _____ HAS A STRUCTURE SIMILAR TO THE
      STEROIDS.
      A. C
      B. B-1
      C. A
      D. D
      E. K

1794.   _____ IS A SYNTHETIC FORM OF VITAMIN K.
      A. Calciferol
      B. Tocopherol
      C. Biotin
      D. Menadione
      E. Cholesterol

1795.   ACTH IS SECRETED BY THE:
A. Liver
B. Thyroid
C. Pituitary
D. Isles of Langerhans
E. Parathyroid

1796.   DRUGS CONTAINING HYDROXYL OR CARBOXYL GROUPS
ARE DETOXIFIED BY:
A. Hippuric acid
B. Glucuronic acid
C. Acetylation
D. Reduction
E. Hydrolysis

1797.   BREAKING DOWN OF MASSIVE PARTICLES TO A SIZE IN THE
COLLOIDAL RANGE IS CALLED:
A. Tyndallization
B. Peptization
C. Pasteurization
D. Levigation
E. Trituration

1798.   PASSIVE DIFFUSION REQUIRES _____ ENERGY.
A. No   D. Kinetic
B. High   E. Electrical
C. Low

1799.   BLOOD PLATELETS ARE ALSO KNOWN AS:
A. Leukocytes
B. Erythrocytes
C. Thrombocytes
D. Phagocytes
E. Reticulocytes

1800.   _____ DRUGS ARE ABSORBED MAINLY FROM THE STOMACH.
A. Alkaline   D. All
B. Neutral   E. No
C. Acidic

1801.   THE NUCLEIC ACIDS, RNA AND DNA, PLAY IMPORTANT ROLES
IN THE BIOSYNTHESIS OF PROTEIN. A SUGAR INHERENT IN
THEIR STRUCTURES IS:
A. Glucose   D. Sorbose
B. Sucrose   E. None of these
C. Fructose

1802.   AN IMPORTANT INITIAL STEP IN THE BIOSYNTHESIS OF
PROTEINS INVOLVES:
A. Amino acid incorporation into peptides
B. Incorporation of thymine into DNA
C. Hydrolysis of RNA by ribonuclease
D. Combination of amino acids with DNA
E. "Activation" of amino acids

1803. GLYCOGENESIS TAKES PLACE MAINLY IN THE:
    A. Pancreas   D. Spleen
    B. Blood   E. Liver
    C. Intestine

1804. AN IMPORTANT PROTEIN AMINO ACID IS THE HORMONE THYROXIN
    WHICH IS PROBABLY SYNTHESIZED FROM:
    A. Tyrosine   D. Iodine monochloride
    B. Indole-5, 6-quinine   E. None of these
    C. Adrenochrome

1805. IT HAS BEEN SHOWN THAT AN IMPORTANT STEP IN THE META-
    BOLISM OF EPINEPHRINE AND NOREPINEPHRINE IS:
    A. Oxidation of the amino group by cytochrome oxidase
    B. Reduction of the side chain
    C. Hydrolysis of the amino group
    D. O-methylation
    E. Oxidation of the catechol nucleus

1806. 3,4-DIHYDROXYPHENYLALANINE (DOPA) HAS BEEN SHOWN TO BE
    THE PRECURSOR OF BOTH:
    A. Tyrosine and alanine
    B. Norepinephrine and glycine
    C. Thyroxin and adrenalin
    D. Melanin and norepinephrine
    E. None of these

1807. _____ NEURONS TRANSMIT IMPULSES FROM SENSORY TO
    MOTOR NEURONS.
    A. Afferent   D. Internuncial
    B. Glial   E. Efferent
    C. Microglia

1808. SOME TISSUES FORM LACTIC ACID UNDER AEROBIC CONDITIONS;
    THIS PHENOMENON, ESPECIALLY CHARACTERISTIC OF TUMOR
    TISSUES, IS TERMED:
    A. Aerobic glycolysis   D. Oxidative-phosphorylation
    B. Lactation   E. None of these
    C. Oxidation

1809. THE PYRIDINE NUCLEOTIDES, DPN AND TPN, ARE ESSENTIAL
    CO-FACTORS IN THE METABOLISM OF MANY SUBSTANCES. AN
    IMPORTANT PART OF THE STRUCTURE OF THESE MOLECULES IS:
    A. Vitamin A   D. Vitamin E
    B. Vitamin C   E. All of these
    C. Nicotinamide

1810. IN ACTIVE TRANSPORT, A (AN) _____ SUBSTANCE IS REQUIRED.
    A. Acidic
    B. Alkaline
    C. Neutral
    D. Charged
    E. Carrier

1811.   FOR THE COMPLETE OXIDATION OF A GLUCOSYL UNIT OF
        GLYCOGEN DOWN THROUGH THE CITRIC ACID CYCLE, HOW
        MANY "ENERGY RICH" BONDS IN THE FORM OF ATP ARE
        PRODUCED?
        A. 12   D. 39
        B. 35   E. None of these
        C. 30

1812.   AN IMPORTANT VITAMIN NECESSARY FOR PYRUVIC ACID
        OXIDATION IS:
        A. Vitamin A
        B. Vitamin D
        C. Vitamins A and D
        D. Thiamine hydrochloride
        E. Vitamin B6

1813.   THE INCIDENCE OF SIDE EFFECTS FROM L-DOPA APPROACHES
        _____%.
        A. 25%   D. 100%
        B. 50%   E. None of these
        C. 75%

1814.   AEROBIC OXIDATION OF CARBOHYDRATES IS MEDIATED VIA:
        A. The urea cycle
        B. The tricarboxylic acid cycle
        C. The pentose phosphate shunt
        D. Embden-Myerhof pathway
        E. All of the above

1815.   WHICH OF THE FOLLOWING WOULD HAVE LITTLE EFFECT ON
        RATE OF ABSORPTION OF A DRUG?
        A. Strength
        B. pH
        C. Active transport
        D. Particle size
        E. Crystalline form

1816.   PHENYTOIN CAUSES ELEVATED BLOOD GLUCOSE LEVELS BY:
        A. Enhancing degradation of insulin
        B. Increasing glucose absorption
        C. Increasing glucagon release
        D. Decreasing insulin release
        E. B and C

1817.   WHICH IS A GOOD DIAGNOSTIC FOR BRONCHOGRAPHY?
        A. Phenol red
        B. Barium sulfate
        C. Decholin
        D. Propyliodone (Dionosil)
        E. Fluoroscein

1818.   MOST "NORMAL VALUES" IN URINALYSIS ARE BASED ON:
         A. mg or Gm per 100 ml
         B. Gm per liter
         C. mg %
         D. Gm per 24 hour excretion
         E. None of the above

1819.   _____ IS DESTROYED BY PROTEOLYTIC ENZYMES WHEN
         GIVEN ORALLY.
         A. Prednisone   D. ACTH
         B. Prednisolone   E. Dexamethasone
         C. Methylprednisone

1820.   AN AMINO ACID USED TO SWEETEN NONCALORIC BEVERAGES IS:
         A. Glycine
         B. Phenylalanine
         C. Histidine
         D. Valine
         E. Methionine

FOR EACH OF THE FOLLOWING MULTIPLE CHOICE QUESTIONS
SELECT THE ONE MOST APPROPRIATE ANSWER:

1821.   A PATIENT IN A DIABETIC COMA:
A. May have the odor of acetone on his breath
B. May be perspiring profusely
C. Usually recovers without treatment
D. May twitch excessively
E. None of the above

1822.   ONE OF THE MOST POTENT STIMULANTS OF THE RESPIRATORY
CENTER IS:
A. Increased pO_2 in the blood
B. A decreased pO_2 in the blood
C. An increased pCO_2 in the blood
D. A decreased pCO_2 in the blood
E. None of these

1823.   A SUBSTANCE PRESENT IN THE SMALL INTESTINE WHICH INHIBITS
GASTRIC SECRETION IS:
A. Enterokinin   D. Enterokinase
B. Histamine   E. None of these
C. Enterogastrone

1824.   ONE OF THE PHYSIOLOGICAL EFFECTS OF AN INCREASED CO_2
IN THE BLOOD IS:
A. Increased dissociation of oxyhemoglobin
B. Increased mental activity
C. Decreased respiration
D. Decreased dissociation of oxyhemoglobin
E. None of these

1825.   METABOLIC ACIDOSIS MAY BE BROUGHT ABOUT BY:
A. Loss of CO_2 by increased ventilation
B. Retention of CO_2 brought about by respiratory obstruction
C. Persistent vomiting
D. Absorption of excessive amounts of $NaHCO_3$
E. None of these

1826.   XEROSTOMIA IS:
A. Loss of night vision   D. Dryness of mouth
B. Decreased peripheral vision E. Loss of taste
C. Muscle twitching

1827.   THE P WAVE OF THE ELECTROCARDIOGRAM IS ASSOCIATED WITH:
A. Auricular repolarization
B. Auricular contraction
C. Auricular depolarization
D. Ventricular repolarization
E. None of these

1828.   ONE OF THE FACTORS REQUIRED FOR THE MATURATION OF THE
        RED BLOOD CELL IS:
        A. Vitamin A   D. Vitamin E
        B. Vitamin D   E. None of these
        C. Vitamin B$_{12}$

1829.   THE A WAVE OF THE VENOUS PULSE IS CAUSED BY:
        A. Auricular contraction which impedes blood flow in the large veins
        B. Incoming blood which stagnates during ventricular systole
        C. The thrust of blood into the aorta which is transmitted to the large
            veins
        D. An abnormally constricted vena cava
        E. None of these

1830.   THE DISINTEGRATION OF THE PLATELETS GIVES RISE TO A FACTOR
        REQUIRED FOR NORMAL BLOOD COAGULATION:
        A. Thromboplastin   D. Fibrinogen
        B. Thrombin   E. None of these
        C. Prothrombin

1831.   A CONDITION IN WHICH THERE IS A DECREASE IN URINE EXCRETION
        IS CALLED:
        A. Anuria   D. Uropenia
        B. Polyuria   E. Cytosuria
        C. Oliguria

1832.   THE EFFECTS OF VAGAL STIMULATION ON THE HEART ARE
        INDUCED AT ONCE; AN EFFECT NOT PRODUCED IS:
        A. Slower cardiac rate
        B. Weaker auricular contraction
        C. Depression of the A-V node
        D. Shorter refractory period of auricular muscle
        E. None of these

1833.   CONTRACTION OF THE HEART IS INITIATED BY THE:
        A. SA node
        B. AV node
        C. Bundles of His
        D. Left atrium
        E. Right ventricle

1834.   DRUGS WHICH STIMULATE THE PARASYMPATHETIC BRANCH OF
        THE AUTONOMIC NERVOUS SYSTEM ARE CALLED:
        A. Anticholinergics
        B. Adrenergic agents
        C. Cholinergic agents
        D. Cholinolytic agents
        E. Sympathomimetics

1835.   THE TOTAL QUANTITY OF AIR THAT CAN BE EXPELLED FROM THE
        LUNGS FOLLOWING A MAXIMAL INSPIRATION IS KNOWN AS THE:
        A. Vital capacity
        B. Tidal volume
        C. Expiratory reserve volume
        D. Functional residual capacity
        E. None of these

1836.   THE RESPIRATORY CENTER IS LOCATED IN THE:
        A. Cerebrum   D. Medulla
        B. Cerebellum   E. Pons
        C. Hypothalamus

1837.   THE PRINCIPLE BY WHICH STIMULATION OF ONE MUSCLE CAUSES
        INHIBITION OF AN ANTAGONISTIC MUSCLE IS:
        A. Reciprocal innervation
        B. Peripheral utilization
        C. Unconscious antagonism
        D. Protective accommodation
        E. None of these

1838.   ISOMETRIC CONTRACTION OF MUSCLE IS ASSOCIATED WITH ALL
        OF THE FOLLOWING, EXCEPT:
        A. An action potential   D. Shortening
        B. Tension   E. Production of lactic acid
        C. Heat

1839.   WHEN A SERIES OF REPETITIVE STIMULI ARE APPLIED WITH A
        RATE HIGH ENOUGH TO CAUSE SUMMATION OF CONTRACTION,
        THE MUSCLE IS SAID TO BE IN A STATE OF:
        A. Rigor   D. Fatigue
        B. Tetanus   E. None of these
        C. Irreversible contracture

1840.   IN YOUNG ADULTS NORMAL BLOOD PRESSURE IS:
        A. 100/60
        B. 80/80
        C. 140/90
        D. 120/120
        E. 120/80

1841.   A DRUG USED EXPERIMENTALLY TO DIFFERENTIATE THE END-
        PLATE POTENTIAL FROM THE MUSCLE ACTION POTENTIAL IS:
        A. Epinephrine   D. Curare
        B. Histamine   E. None of these
        C. Creatine phosphate

1842.   SYSTEMIC DIASTOLIC PRESSURE DEPENDS LARGELY UPON:
        A. Cardiac output
        B. Elasticity of vessel walls
        C. Peripheral resistance
        D. A and B
        E. B and C

1843. THE GLOMERULUS IS:
A. A network of capillaries
B. A lymph node
C. A large artery entering the kidney
D. A dilator substance produced by the kidney
E. None of these

1844. HENLE'S LOOP IS FOUND IN THE:
A. Liver   D. Kidney
B. Stomach   E. Inner ear
C. Intestine

1845. _____ IS A LACK OF SPEECH COORDINATION.
A. Dysphasia
B. Paresthesia
C. Dyspnea
D. Diplopia
E. Dyspraxia

1846. BODY SURFACE IS CLOSELY RELATED TO:
A. Volume   D. Age
B. Height   E. All of these
C. Weight

1847. THE TEMPERATURE REGULATING CENTER OF THE BODY IS
IN THE:
A. Medulla
B. Cerebrum
C. Spinal cord
D. Thalamus
E. None of these

1848. THE EFFECT OF ADRENOCORTICAL HORMONE ON THE
KIDNEY IS:
A. Increases the rate of sodium resorption and potassium excretion
B. Decreases the rate of sodium resorption and potassium excretion
C. Increases the rate of sodium and potassium resorption
D. Decreases the rate of sodium and potassium resorption
E. None of these

1849. _____ ARE THE MACROPHAGES OF CNS TISSUE.
A. Microglia
B. Neurilemma
C. Arachnoid villi
D. Folia
E. Microsoma

1850. THE FUNDAMENTAL UNIT OF ORGANIZED NEURAL ACTIVITY IS
THE _____.
A. Ganglion
B. Reflex arc
C. Synapse
D. Afferent neuron
E. Efferent neuron

1851.   A SUBSTANCE USED TO MEASURE THE GLOMERULAR
         FILTRATION RATE IS:
         A. Insulin
         B. Inulin
         C. Diodrast
         D. Para-aminohippuric acid
         E. None of these

1852.   THE ANTIDIURETIC HORMONE IS SECRETED FROM:
         A. Kidney cortex   D. Posterior pituitary
         B. Kidney medulla   E. None of these
         C. Anterior pituitary

1853.   THE EFFECT OF THE ANTIDIURETIC HORMONE IS TO:
         A. Decrease water loss by the lungs
         B. Increase perspiration
         C. Decrease the rate of resorption of water by the kidney
         D. Increase the rate of resorption of water by the kidney
         E. None of these

1854.   THE SYMPATHETIC GANGLIA ARE LOCATED:
         A. Near the heart
         B. Near the spinal cord
         C. Near the adrenal glands
         D. Near the tissues they innervate
         E. In the extremities

1855.   THE CARDIAC RESERVE IS:
         A. The maximal percentage increase in cardiac output that can occur
         B. The amount of blood remaining in the heart after systole
         C. The volume of blood the heart can hold
         D. The volume of blood within the walls of the cardiac musculature that
             can be called upon in an emergency
         E. None of these

1856.   A SUBSTANCE GENERALLY USED FOR MEASURING RENAL PLASMA
         FLOW IS:
         A. Ethyl alcohol   D. Glucose
         B. Inulin   E. None of these
         C. Para-aminohippuric acid

1857.   THE ENDOCRINE GLANDS DIFFER FROM ORDINARY GLANDS BE-
         CAUSE:
         A. They are larger
         B. They are smaller
         C. They secrete substances
         D. They all have the same shape
         E. They are ductless

1858.   THE CHEMICAL MEDIATOR RELEASED AT THE END OF THE
        PARASYMPATHETIC NERVE FIBER IS:
        A. Acetylcholine esterase
        B. Acetylcholine
        C. Epinephrine
        D. Norepinephrine
        E. Amine oxidase

1859.   AN ENDOCRINE GLAND THAT PLAYS AN IMPORTANT ROLE IN
        CALCIUM METABOLISM IS:
        A. Pancreas   D. Parathyroid
        B. Hypophysis   E. Gonads
        C. Thyroid

1860.   ACTIVATED PANCREATIC JUICE CONTAINS:
        A. Trypsin   D. Sodium bicarbonate
        B. Steapsin   E. All of these
        C. Amylopsin

1861.   THE QUANTITY OF HEMOGLOBIN IN 100 ML OF BLOOD AVERAGES:
        A.   5 gm   D. 20 gm
        B. 10 gm   E. None of these
        C. 15 gm

1862.   THE TERM HEMATOCRIT MEANS:
        A. The percentage of the blood that is red blood cells
        B. The percentage of the blood that is plasma
        C. The percentage of the blood volume to the extracellular space
        D. The percentage of new blood formed every 120 days
        E. None of the above

1863.   THE MOST IMPORTANT FUNCTIONAL PROCESS THAT THE
        NEUTROPHILS AND MONOCYTES CARRY OUT IS:
        A. Phagocytosis
        B. IDK
        C. Tachyphylaxis
        D. Urea absorption
        E. None of the above

1864.   THE UPPERMOST PORTION OF THE INTESTINE IS THE:
        A. Cecum
        B. Jejunum
        C. Ileum
        D. Duodenum
        E. Colon

1865.   THE PIGMENT WHICH GIVES THE URINE ITS COLOR IS:
        A. Urochrome
        B. Bilirubin
        C. Biliverdin
        D. Urobilin
        E. None of the above

MATCH THE FOLLOWING SUBSTANCES WITH THE ORGAN OR
GLAND SECRETING EACH:

1866. ___ Epinephrine	A.	Anterior pituitary
1867. ___ Lactogenic hormone	B.	Adrenals
1868. ___ Insulin	C.	Pancreas
1869. ___ Thyroxine	D.	Stomach mucosa
1870. ___ Gastrin	E.	Thyroid
1871. ___ Testosterone		
1872. ___ ACTH		

1873. COR PULMONALE IS:
   A. Obstruction of the lung
   B. Decrease in RBC
   C. Hypertrophy of the right ventricle
   D. Decrease in WBC
   E. Increase in WBC

MATCH THE FOLLOWING:

1874. ___ Principle of divergence	A.	Contraction without external
1875. ___ Principle of convergence		shortening
1876. ___ Stretch reflex	B.	Shortening under constant tension
1877. ___ Crossed extensor reflex	C.	Synaptic innervation of a number
1878. ___ Isometric contraction		of cells by one fiber
1879. ___ Isotonic contraction	D.	Overlapping synaptic innervation
1880. ___ Fasciculation		of one cell by a number of fibers
	E.	Spontaneous intermittent involun-
		tary activity of nervous system
	F.	Active resistance of a muscle
		when pull is exerted upon the
		tendon
	G.	The contralateral accompaniment
		of the flexor reflex

MATCH THE FOLLOWING CONDITIONS WITH THE PART OF THE
BODY EACH IS MOST FREQUENTLY ASSOCIATED WITH:

1881. ___ Hiccup	A.	Stomach
1882. ___ Caries	B.	Diaphragm
1883. ___ Colitis	C.	Skin
1884. ___ Ulcers	D.	Teeth
1885. ___ Urticaria	E.	Intestines

1886. EQUALIZATION OF AIR PRESSURE BETWEEN THE TYMPANIC
   CAVITY AND THE OUTSIDE ATMOSPHERE IS DONE BY THE:
   A. Stapes
   B. Cochlea
   C. Eustachian tube
   D. Anvil
   E. Semicircular canal

1887.   THERE ARE _____ PAIRS OF SPINAL NERVES.
        A. 24   D. 20
        B. 31   E. 10
        C. 36

1888.   THE _____ OF THE SPINAL CORD SERVES AS A CONDUCTING
        PATHWAY FOR IMPULSES.
        A. Gray matter
        B. White matter
        C. Cerebrospinal fluid
        D. Pia mater
        E. Arachnoid

1889.   FIBRINOGEN IS SYNTHESIZED MAINLY IN THE:
        A. Blood
        B. Pancreas
        C. Kidney
        D. Liver
        E. Lung

1890.   _____ IS ESSENTIAL FOR PROTHROMBIN FORMATION.
        A. Vitamin K
        B. Vitamin B-12
        C. Folic acid
        D. Heme
        E. All of the above

1891.   THE NEURO-TRANSMITTER RELEASED AT THE END OF THE
        SYMPATHETIC NERVE FIBER IS:
        A. Epinephrine
        B. Norepinephrine
        C. Acetylcholine
        D. Acetylcholine esterase
        E. Amine oxidase

1892.   DRUGS WHICH CAUSE DILATION OF THE EYE PUPIL ARE:
        A. Miotics
        B. Mydriatics
        C. Cycloplegics
        D. Antispasmodics
        E. Anorectics

1893.   THE MOST COMMON BLOOD TYPE IS:
        A. A   D. AB
        B. B   E. X
        C. O

1894.   ADDISON'S DISEASE IS CAUSED BY DYSFUNCTION OF:
        A. Posterior pituitary
        B. Adrenal medulla
        C. Adrenal cortex
        D. Parathyroids
        E. Bone marrow

1895.   FEVER DURING INFECTION IS DUE TO:
A. Increased heat production, followed by decreased heat loss
B. Decreased heat loss, followed by increased heat production
C. An action of bacterial pyrogens independent of the body's heat-control mechanisms
D. A functional hyperthyroidism due to irritation of the thyroid and release of colloid
E. None of the above

MATCH EACH OF THE FOLLOWING SUBSTANCES WITH THE PHYSIOLOGICAL ITEM OR FUNCTION WHICH IT IS USED TO MEASURE:

A. Plasma volume
B. Total body water
C. Glomerular filtration rate
D. Renal plasma flow
E. Gastric secretion of HCl
F. Conjugating capacity of the liver

1896. ___ PAH
1897. ___ T-1834
1898. ___ Histamine
1899. ___ Inulin
1900. ___ Benzoic acid
1901. ___ Deuterium oxide

1902.   MODERATE STRETCH OF CARDIAC MUSCLE:
A. Strengthens the contractile force
B. Weakens the contractile force
C. Has no effect on the contractile force
D. Abolishes contraction
E. Initiates contraction

1903.   THE O_2 DISSOCIATION CURVE OF HEMOGLOBIN IS SHIFTED TO THE RIGHT BY:
A. Decreased CO_2
B. Increased CO_2
C. Increased pH
D. Increased N_2 tension
E. Decreased N_2 tension

MATCH THE FOLLOWING:

A. Anoxic anoxia
B. Stagnant anoxia
C. Anemic anoxia
D. Histotoxic anoxia

1904. ___ Anoxia due to respiratory obstruction
1905. ___ Anoxia due to cyanide poisoning
1906. ___ Anoxia due to congestive failure
1907. ___ Anoxia due to carbon monoxide poisoning
1908. ___ Anoxia due to low atmospheric oxygen

MATCH EACH OF THE FOLLOWING WITH A FUNCTION EACH
PERFORMS IN THE BODY:

A. Oxygen transport
B. Defense against infection
C. Regulation of pressure
D. Nutrition of fetus
E. Regulates heart rate
F. Balance
G. Electrical transmitter
H. Night vision

1909. ___ Labyrinth
1910. ___ Rods
1911. ___ Umbilical cord
1912. ___ Hemoglobin
1913. ___ W. B. C.
1914. ___ Carotid sinus
1915. ___ Vagus
1916. ___ AV node

1917.   THE BUNDLES OF HIS ARE FOUND IN THE:
A. Lung
B. Intestines
C. Liver
D. Heart
E. Kidney

1918.   THE PACEMAKER OF THE HEART IS THE:
A. Coronary artery
B. Right ventricle
C. SA node
D. AV node
E. Left ventricle

1919.   THE CHIEF DANGER OF ANY DRUG CAUSING RESPIRATORY
STIMULATION IS:
A. Liver damage
B. The chance of inducing convulsions
C. Kidney damage
D. Induction of hypotension
E. Induction of hypertension

1920.   WHICH OF THE FOLLOWING SUBSTANCES IS THE SOURCE OF
ENERGY IN NERVE FIBERS?
A. Potassium
B. Sodium ion
C. Calcium ion
D. Glucose
E. Magnesium ion

1921.   RALES ARE:
A. Lesions
B. Visual disturbances
C. Flashing pains
D. Abnormal chest sounds
E. None of the above

1922.   THERE ARE_____PAIRS OF CRANIAL NERVES.
        A. 8
        B. 10
        C. 12
        D. 14
        E. 16

1923.   WHICH OF THE FOLLOWING IS NOT NORMALLY FILTERED OR
        REABSORBED TO A SIGNIFICANT DEGREE?
        A. Para-aminohippurate   D. Plasma proteins
        B. Inulin   E. NaCl
        C. Xylose

1924.   WHICH OF THE FOLLOWING SUBSTANCES IS FILTERED BUT NOT
        REABSORBED BY THE TUBULES?
        A. Xylose   D. NaCl
        B. Plasma proteins   E. Para-aminohippurate
        C. Inulin

1925.   THE DIFFUSION OF CO_2 ACROSS THE ALVEOLAR MEMBRANE IS
        20 TIMES FASTER THAN THAT OF O_2 BECAUSE:
        A. CO_2 is actively transferred
        B. The alveolar area available for CO_2 diffusion is larger
        C. CO_2 is more soluble in H_2O (than is O_2) which enables it to pass the
           membrane with greater readiness
        D. The CO_2 pressure gradient is larger
        E. None of these

1926.   THE PRINCIPAL ACTION OF LYMPH GLANDS IS:
        A. To destroy microorganisms   D. To filter out solids
        B. As a warning system   E. None of these
        C. To reduce fever

1927.   DIVERTICULOSIS IS USUALLY ASSOCIATED WITH THE:
        A. Stomach
        B. Small intestine
        C. Liver
        D. Skin
        E. Colon

1928.   THE SENSORY GANGLION OF THE BRAIN STEM IS THE:
        A. Cerebral cortex   D. Medulla
        B. Hypothalamus   E. Basal ganglia
        C. Thalamus

1929.   PREDISPOSING FACTORS TO PEPTIC ULCER ARE:
        A. Endocrine disorders
        B. Genetic influence
        C. Emotional disturbances
        D. B and C
        E. All of the above

1930. WHEN LIGHT RAYS COME TO A FOCUS BEHIND THE RETINA, THE
       EYE IS SAID TO BE:
       A. Hypermetropic   D. Myopic
       B. Presbyopic   E. Emmetropic
       C. Astigmatic

1931. PROGRESSIVE FIBROSIS AND SCARRING OF THE LIVER IS KNOWN
       AS:
       A. Diverticulitis   D. Cirrhosis
       B. Diverticulosis   E. Ulcerative colitis
       C. Hepatitis

1932. WHICH OF THE FOLLOWING IS NOT ONE OF THE CARDINAL META-
       BOLIC EFFECTS OF THE PARATHYROID HORMONE?
       A. Hyperphosphaturia   D. Hyperphosphatemia
       B. Hypercalciuria   E. Hypercalcemia
       C. Hypophosphatemia

1933. THE COUGH CENTER IS LOCATED IN THAT PORTION OF THE BRAIN
       CALLED THE:
       A. Temporal lobe   D. Cerebellum
       B. Medulla   E. Cerebrum
       C. Thalamus

1934. ALCOHOL IS DETOXIFIED MAINLY BY THE:
       A. Lung
       B. Gallbladder
       C. Kidney
       D. Liver
       E. Stomach

1935. THE FIRST HEART SOUND IS THE RESULT OF:
       A. The closure of the semilunar valves
       B. Closure of the auriculoventricular valves
       C. The rapid inflow of blood from auricle into ventricle
       D. Inflow of blood from ventricle into the aorta
       E. None of the above

1936. PARIETAL CELLS SECRETE:
       A. Sodium bicarbonate   D. Bile salts
       B. Hydrochloric acid   E. ACTH
       C. Insulin

1937. THE RESPIRATORY STIMULANT EFFECT OF CO_2 IS DUE TO A
       DIRECT ACTION ON THE:
       A. Carotid body
       B. Carotid sinus
       C. Aortic body
       D. Respiratory center
       E. None of the above

1938. THE ION IN HIGHEST CONCENTRATION IN THE CELLS IS:
A. Na   D. Ca
B. Mg   E. Fe
C. K

1939. THE ION IN HIGHEST CONCENTRATION OUTSIDE THE CELL IS:
A. Na   D. Ca
B. Mg   E. Fe
C. K

1940. HEAVY METALS EXERT THEIR TOXIC EFFECTS IN THE BODY BY:
A. Blocking enzymes
B. Sclerosing tissues
C. Precipitating proteins
D. Depressing oxygen exchange
E. None of the above

1941. A TERM DENOTING DRYNESS OF THE MOUTH IS:
A. Zerophthalmia   D. Xerotocia
B. Stomatitis   E. Xeromenia
C. Xerostomia

1942. POLYCYTHEMIA IS CHARACTERIZED BY:
A. Anemia
B. High W. B. C.
C. High R. B. C.
D. Low R. B. C.
E. Eosinophilia

1943. THE MOST IMPORTANT CARDIAC AND VASOMOTOR CENTERS
ARE SITUATED IN THE:
A. Hypothalamus   D. Cerebellum
B. Medulla   E. None of these
C. Cerebrum

1944. MOST OF THE VENOUS CO_2 IS IN THE FORM OF:
A. Carbonate   D. Dissolved CO_2
B. Carbonic acid   E. None of these
C. Bicarbonate

1945. A SUDDEN INCREASE IN ARTERIAL BLOOD PRESSURE CAUSES:
A. An increase in heart rate
B. A fall in venous pressure
C. Reflex bradycardia
D. Reflex hyperpnea
E. Reflex increase in venous pressure

1946. _____ IS A HORMONE RELEASED BY THE PRESENCE OF
FAT IN THE DUODENUM AND CAUSES CONTRACTION OF GALLBLAD-
DER MUSCLE.
A. Secretin   D. Corticotropin
B. Pancreolipase   E. Gonadotropin
C. Cholecystokinin

1947.   THE pH OF THE BLOOD IS THE pH OF:
   A.   The cells
   B.   The plasma
   C.   The average of cell and plasma
   D.   The difference between cell and plasma
   E.   None of the above

1948.   BILIRUBIN IS PRODUCED BY:
   A.   Biosynthesis   D.   Decomposition of bile salts
   B.   The kidney   E.   The spleen
   C.   Hemoglobin decomposition

1949.   THE _____ TRANSPORT(S) URINE TO THE BLADDER.
   A.   Urethra   D.   Loop of Henle
   B.   Ureters   E.   None of these
   C.   Glomeruli

1950.   RETROPERITONEAL MEANS:
   A.   In front of the peritoneum
   B.   Behind the peritoneum
   C.   On the right side of the peritoneum
   D.   On the left side of the peritoneum
   E.   Near the peritoneum

1951.   THE NORMAL R.Q. OF MAN UNDER RESTING CONDITIONS IS:
   A.   0.92   D.   1.7
   B.   0.72   E.   None of these
   C.   0.82

1952.   A SELECTIVE LOSS OF EXTRACELLULAR ELECTROLYTE
        WITHOUT WATER RESULTS IN:
   A.   Overexpansion of the extracellular fluid volume with dehydration
        of cells
   B.   Anhydremia and cellular hydration
   C.   Hydremia and cellular hydration
   D.   Anhydremia and cellular dehydration
   E.   None of the above

1953.   IF ALL OTHER FACTORS REMAIN CONSTANT, THE VELOCITY
        OF BLOOD FLOW IN THE AORTA IS:
   A.   Greater than the pulse wave velocity
   B.   Approximately equal to the pulse wave velocity
   C.   Inversely proportional to aortic diameter
   D.   Directly proportional to the square of the aortic diameter
   E.   Independent of the left ventricular minute volume

1954.   VINCENT'S ANGINA IS A DISEASE OF THE:
   A.   Heart
   B.   Coronary artery
   C.   Veins
   D.   Mouth
   E.   None of the above

1955.   DYSPHAGIA IS DEFINED AS:
         A. Earache from any cause
         B. Painful menstruation
         C. Toothache
         D. Difficulty in swallowing
         E. Painful eye inflammation

FOR QUESTIONS 1956-1965 USE THE FOLLOWING KEY TO ANSWER
EACH QUESTION:

         A. Raises, increases or elevates
         B. Lowers, depresses or decreases
         C. Has no effect on.

1956. ___ Effect of epinephrine on blood pressure.

1957. ___ Effect of morphine on size of the eye pupil.

1958. ___ Effect of edecrin on potassium levels.

1959. ___ Effect of dehydration on urine output.

1960. ___ Effect of atropine on salivary secretions.

1961. ___ Effect of bile salts on absorption.

1962. ___ Effect of infections on WBC.

1963. ___ Effect of MAO inhibitors on serotonin levels.

1964. ___ Effect of morphine on bowel movements.

1965. ___ Effect of iron on WBC.

1966.   THE SINOATRIAL NODE IS STIMULATED BY:
         A. The myogenic reflex
         B. The preganglionic sympathetic endings
         C. The postganglionic sympathetic endings
         D. The preganglionic parasympathetic endings
         E. None of these

1967.   THE RESPIRATORY QUOTIENT IS:
        A. Volume O_2 inhaled/volume O_2 exhaled
        B. Volume CO_2 inhaled/volume CO_2 exhaled
        C. Volume CO_2 produced/volume O_2 absorbed
        D. Volume O_2 produced/volume CO_2 absorbed
        E. None of the above

1968.   _____ IS A SUDDEN ATTACK OF CONVULSIONS NOT OF
        CENTRAL ORIGIN.
        A. Eccyesis   D. Eclampsia
        B. Ecchymosis   E. Eburnation
        C. Ecmnesia

1969.   DISCS ARE ASSOCIATED WITH THE:
        A. Brain   D. Arms
        B. Feet   E. Taste buds
        C. Spinal column

1970.   MIC IS THE ABBREVIATION FOR:
        A. Minimum intercostal cleavage
        B. Minimum intracellular concentration
        C. Maximum intracellular concentration
        D. Minimum inhibitory concentration
        E. Maximum inhibitory concentration

1971.   TETANY IN HYPOPARATHYROIDISM IS CAUSED BY:
        A. High pH of serum   D. Low calcium
        B. High calcium   E. High phosphorus
        C. Low phosphorus

1972.   METHYL TESTOSTERONE IS A HORMONE OF THE:
        A. Corpus luteum   D. Pituitary
        B. Follicle   E. Placenta
        C. Interstitial cells

        MATCH THE FOLLOWING:

1973. ___ Somatotropin   A. Parathyroid
1974. ___ Vasopressin   B. Anterior pituitary
1975. ___ Oxytocin   C. Posterior pituitary
1976. ___ Aldosterone   D. Adrenal cortex
1977. ___ Progesterone   E. Adrenal medulla
1978. ___ Glucagon   F. Placenta
1979. ___ Thyrotropin   G. Corpus luteum
1980. ___ Secretin   H. Beta cells of pancreas
1981. ___ ACTH   I. Alpha cells of pancreas
1982. ___ Parathormone   J. None of these
1983. ___ FSH
1984. ___ Chorionic gonadotropin
1985. ___ Insulin

1986.   ESTRADIOL IS A HORMONE OF THE:
        A. Follicle
        B. Anterior pituitary
        C. Cells of Leydig
        D. Seminal vesicles
        E. None of these

1987. SECRETION OF ADRENAL CORTICAL HORMONES IS PRIMARILY
CONTROLLED BY:
A. Somatotropic hormone   D. ACTH
B. Epinephrine   E. ICSH
C. Glucagon

1988. MOST PATIENTS SUFFER FROM ACUTE RENAL FAILURE AS A RESULT
OF:
A. Dehydration   D. Bacterial infection
B. Nitrosis   E. Hyperkalemia
C. Cirrhosis

1989. THE ADRENAL STEROID HYDROCORTISONE'S ACTION IS PRIMARILY
CONCERNED WITH:
A. Water balance   D. Basal metabolism
B. Salt metabolism   E. Calcium metabolism
C. Carbohydrate metabolism

1990. GAMMA GLOBULIN IS:
A. A protein fraction of the blood
B. The portion of the blood that may be removed by centrifuging
C. The part of the blood removed by the clot
D. The part of the blood that is soluble in trichloracetic acid
E. The part of the blood that cannot be salted out with ammonium sulfate

1991. THE PART OF THE EYE THAT IS CONCERNED WITH NIGHT VISION
IS (ARE) THE:
A. Cones   D. Lens
B. Rods   E. Eye muscle
C. Iris

1992. THE LUNG IS COVERED BY THE:
A. Bronchioles   D. Alveoli
B. Alveolar sac   E. Cartilage
C. Pleura

1993. THE SYMPATHETIC SYSTEM RECEIVES ITS CONNECTION WITH THE
CENTRAL NERVOUS SYSTEM FROM WHICH AREA?
A. Cranial nerves   D. Lumbar spinal cord
B. Thoracic spinal cord   E. Lumbo-pelvic spinal cord
C. Thoracolumbar spinal cord

1994. WHICH ONE OF THE FOLLOWING PERCENTAGES REPRESENTS THE
EXTRACELLULAR PORTION OF TOTAL BODY WATER?
A. Approximately 33%
B. Approximately 20%
C. Approximately 50%
D. Approximately 75%
E. Approximately 10%

1995. _____ IS INFLAMMATION OF THE KIDNEY SUBSTANCE AND
PELVIS.
A. Pyelonephritis   D. Pyometritis
B. Hepatitis   E. Perichondritis
C. Pyemesis

1996. THE ELECTROCARDIOGRAM REVEALS THE TIME OF CONDUCTION
FROM THE SINO-ATRIAL NODE TO THE SUBENDOCARDIAL VENTRI-
CULAR MUSCLE BY THE LENGTH OF:
A. QRS interval   D. P-T interval
B. Q-T interval   E. R-S interval
C. P-R or P-Q interval

1997. THE VILLI ARE FOUND IN THE:
A. Small intestine   D. Esophagus
B. Large intestine   E. None of these
C. Stomach

1998. THE NORMAL DAILY REQUIREMENT OF VITAMIN D IN A CHILD IS:
A. 200 units   D. 2000 units
B. 800 units   E. 2500 units
C. 1400 units

1999. ALL BUT ONE OF THE FOLLOWING FACTORS CAUSES CONSTRICTION
OF THE CAPILLARIES:
A. Decreased temperature   D. Lack of CO_2
B. Lack of H^+ E. Fever
C. Decreased metabolism

2000. _____ IS A WASTING DUE TO LACK OF NUTRITION TO A
BODY PART.
A. Atrophy   D. Hyperplasia
B. Hypertrophy   E. Gerontopia
C. Aphasia

2001. A SPHYGMOMANOMETER IS USED TO MEASURE:
A. Lung capacity
B. Blood pressure
C. Basic metabolic rate
D. Electrical impulses of the heart
E. Temperature

2002. THE HUMAN OVUM HAS _____ CHROMOSOMES.
A. 12   D. 96
B. 24   E. None of these
C. 48

2003. THE LONGEST AND STRONGEST BONE OF THE BODY IS THE:
A. Pelvis   D. Femur
B. Metacarpal   E. Radius
C. Ulna

THE FOLLOWING HEART TONES ARE DUE TO:

2004. ___	First heart sound	A.	Diastolic inrush of blood into the ventricle
2005. ___	Second heart sound		
2006. ___	Third heart sound	B.	Isometric phase of ventricular con-
2007. ___	Fourth heart sound		traction and closure of AV valves
		C.	Contraction of atria
		D.	Closure of arterial valve

RENAL CLEARANCE IS MEASURED BY:

Substance   Function Measured

2008. ___	PAH	A.	Tubular
2009. ___	PAH + inulin	B.	Glomerular
2010. ___	Inulin	C.	Tubular and glomerular

2011.   THE BREAST BONE IS CALLED THE:
A.   Sternum
B.   Thorax
C.   Ribs
D.   Ulna
E.   Femur

2012.   DYSPNEA MEANS:
A.   Painful muscle spasm
B.   Pain in the heart
C.   Pain in extremities
D.   Painful breathing
E.   None of the above

2013.   CYSTITIS IS AN INFLAMMATION OF THE _____.
A.   Ovary
B.   Vagina
C.   Urethra
D.   Kidney
E.   Bladder

2014.   BLOOD MAKES UP ABOUT_____OF BODY WEIGHT.
A.   1/6
B.   1/25
C.   1/13
D.   1/20
E.   1/30

2015.   ADRENAL CORTEX IS ANATOMICALLY COMPOSED OF THE
FOLLOWING ZONES, EXCEPT:
A.   Zona glomerulosa
B.   Zona fasciculata
C.   Zona granularis
D.   Zona reticularis
E.   Zona intermedia

2016.   PITUITARY DWARFISM IS CAUSED BY:
A.   Hypofunction of the eosinophilic cells
B.   Hypofunction of the basophilic cells
C.   Hyperfunction of the eosinophilic cells
D.   Hyperfunction of the basophilic cells
E.   None of the above

2017.   THE LONGEST MUSCLE IN THE BODY IS THE _____
MUSCLE.
A.   Abductor longus
B.   Gluteus maximus
C.   Transversus abdominus
D.   Psoas major
E.   Sartorius

2018.   THE BUNDLE OF HIS IS:
A.   Composed of nerve fibers
B.   Composed of ordinary heart muscle
C.   Made up of muscle fibers adapted to conduct impulses from atria
to ventricles
D.   Innervated by the vagus directly
E.   None of the above

2019.   THE SINO-ATRIAL NODE IS MADE UP OF:
A.   Modified nervous tissue
B.   A special tissue combining the properties of muscle and nerve
C.   Modified cardiac muscle
D.   Ganglionic cells
E.   Smooth muscle

2020.   THERE ARE OVER _____ MUSCLES IN THE HUMAN BODY.
A.   100
B.   200
C.   400
D.   500
E.   700

The author has made every effort to thoroughly verify the answers to the questions which appear on the preceding pages. However, as in any text, some inaccuracies and ambiguities may occur.

THE PUBLISHERS

SECTION I

1. A	46. A	91. B	136. E	181. E	226. C
2. C	47. B	92. A	137. D	182. B	227. E
3. B	48. E	93. A	138. E	183. A	228. D
4. C	49. F	94. D	139. A	184. A	229. I
5. B	50. D	95. B	140. C	185. B	230. D
6. A	51. G	96. C	141. A	186. C	231. A
7. B	52. D	97. B	142. D	187. E	232. G
8. A	53. C	98. E	143. D	188. D	233. H
9. A	54. C	99. C	144. D	189. D	234. E
10. D	55. D	100. C	145. D	190. B	235. B
11. D	56. D	101. A	146. B	191. C	236. C
12. C	57. E	102. A	147. C	192. D	237. F
13. B	58. E	103. A	148. E	193. B	238. J
14. B	59. A	104. B	149. A	194. E	239. H
15. A	60. E	105. B	150. D	195. A	240. F
16. B	61. A	106. E	151. A	196. C	241. C
17. B	62. C	107. E	152. A	197. E	242. J
18. C	63. A	108. B	153. D	198. D	243. D
19. C	64. A	109. C	154. D	199. B	244. E
20. E	65. D	110. A	155. B	200. B	245. B
21. C	66. E	111. E	156. B	201. E	246. I
22. E	67. E	112. D	157. C	202. E	247. A
23. C	68. D	113. A	158. A	203. A	248. G
24. C	69. A	114. A	159. B	204. D	249. D
25. C	70. C	115. D	160. C	205. A	250. D
26. B	71. B	116. C	161. B	206. G	251. C
27. B	72. E	117. B	162. D	207. C	252. D
28. E	73. B	118. C	163. A	208. H	253. D
29. B	74. B	119. C	164. E	209. I	254. B
30. B	75. C	120. A	165. B	210. J	255. A
31. B	76. D	121. A	166. C	211. E	256. C
32. E	77. C	122. D	167. A	212. F	257. E
33. A	78. D	123. B	168. D	213. B	258. B
34. D	79. D	124. A	169. E	214. E	259. D
35. B	80. D	125. A	170. B	215. B	260. A
36. C	81. D	126. B	171. B	216. E	261. B
37. C	82. C	127. C	172. D	217. B	262. B
38. C	83. C	128. C	173. A	218. A	263. B
39. A	84. B	129. A	174. C	219. A	264. C
40. B	85. C	130. C	175. D	220. C	265. B
41. E	86. B	131. E	176. C	221. D	266. A
42. D	87. E	132. C	177. A	222. E	267. D
43. A	88. B	133. A	178. B	223. B	268. E
44. A	89. B	134. C	179. B	224. C	269. C
45. C	90. B	135. B	180. B	225. E	270. B

SECTION I

271. A	324. A	377. C	430. B	483. B	536. D
272. B	325. A	378. E	431. I	484. D	537. C
273. E	326. D	379. A	432. G	485. A	538. D
274. A	327. C	380. B	433. B	486. C	539. B
275. A	328. C	381. B	434. E	487. E	540. E
276. B	329. A	382. B	435. C	488. G	541. A
277. C	330. B	383. C	436. A	489. B	542. A
278. A	331. B	384. A	437. D	490. C	543. D
279. D	332. C	385. E	438. J	491. J	544. B
280. E	333. D	386. C	439. F	492. H ·	545. C
281. E	334. C	387. D	440. H	493. A	546. E
282. C	335. A	388. B	441. A	494. D	547. H
283. B	336. D	389. A	442. C	495. L	548. G
284. D	337. A	390. C	443. C	496. F	549. F
285. A	338. D	391. C	444. C	497. I	550. J
286. C	339. E	392. F	445. D	498. K	551. I
287. B	340. E	393. B	446. A	499. A	552. E
288. A	341. D	394. D	447. E	500. C	553. G
289. D	342. A	395. A	448. C	501. E	554. C
290. E	343. C	396. G	449. F	502. B	555. J
291. C	344. B	397. E	450. B	503. D	556. D
292. A	345. D	398. C	451. E	504. D	557. I
293. E	346. E	399. E	452. D	505. E	558. A
294. A	347. E	400. D	453. C	506. B	559. F
295. B	348. D	401. B	454. A	507. A	560. B
296. E	349. A	402. A	455. F	508. F	561. H
297. A	350. C	403. E	456. B	509. E	562. C
298. C	351. D	404. C	457. I	510. C	563. E
299. D	352. A	405. B	458. H	511. G	564. A
300. C	353. D	406. B	459. K	512. B	565. D
301. D	354. C	407. D	460. G	513. H	566. B
302. B	355. B	408. B	461. L	514. A	567. G
303. E	356. F	409. C	462. J	515. D	568. F
304. A	357. E	410. D	463. B	516. F	569. H
305. C	358. D	411. B	464. E	517. I	570. F
306. D	359. B	412. B	465. C	518. J	571. G
307. A	360. E	413. D	466. J	519. D	572. H
308. D	361. H	414. B	467. F	520. F	573. K
309. A	362. B	415. C	468. A	521. A	574. C
310. E	363. C	416. A	469. G	522. G	575. A
311. C	364. G	417. E	470. D	523. H	576. I
312. D	365. A	418. C	471. I	524. C	577. E
313. B	366. D	419. A	472. H	525. B	578. B
314. C	367. F	420. E	473. C	526. E	579. M
315. E	368. C	421. A	474. C	527. J	580. L
316. G	369. A	422. C	475. E	528. I	581. J
317. A	370. D	423. B	476. F	529. E	582. D
318. H	371. E	424. D	477. A	530. E	583. C
319. B	372. B	425. A	478. B	531. D	584. G
320. F	373. E	426. E	479. D	532. A	585. D
321. J	374. B	427. D	480. A	533. E	586. H
322. D	375. B	428. B	481. B	534. C	587. F
323. I	376. D	429. C	482. D	535. B	588. L

Schering Corporation a diversified organization, dedicated to the discovery and development of quality pharmaceuticals.

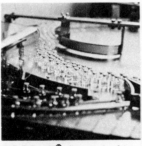

A major portion of Schering's efforts is directed to serving the health professions with outstanding pharmaceuticals. Recent contributions from Schering include DIPROSONE® (brand of betamethasone dipropionate), GARAMYCIN® (brand of gentamicin sulfate, U.S.P.) HYPERSTAT® (brand of diazoxide) and VANCERIL® (brand of beclomethasone dipropionate).

Schering research is also providing improved therapy for inflammatory diseases, allergies, cardiovascular diseases, mental and emotional illnesses, and certain respiratory and endocrine disorders.

SCHERING CORPORATION
Dedicated to Progress in Pharmaceutical Research

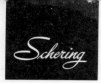

Schering Corporation, World-Wide Facilities To Meet World-Wide Demands.

In the United States—
Laboratories, Plants and Offices in 26 cities in 12 states.

California	Maryland	Tennessee
Florida	Massachusetts	Texas
Georgia	New Jersey	Virginia
Illinois	Ohio	Wisconsin

And around the world—
Represented in 55 cities in 39 countries.

Argentina	Guatemala	Norway
Australia	Hong Kong	Panama
Austria	India	Peru
Belgium	Indonesia	Philippines
Brazil	Iran	Portugal
Canada	Italy	Puerto Rico
Chile	Jamaica	South Africa
Colombia	Japan	Spain
Denmark	Kenya	Sweden
Ecuador	Lebanon	Switzerland
Finland	Mexico	Thailand
France	Netherlands	United Kingdom
Germany	New Zealand	Venezuela

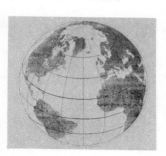

SECTION I

589. A	642. H	695. D	748. D
590. I	643. J	696. E	749. H
591. K	644. L	697. C	750. E
592. B	645. E	698. D	751. C
593. M	646. A	699. B	752. B
594. J	647. C	700. B	753. A
595. E	648. A	701. B	754. B
596. C	649. C	702. C	755. C
597. A	650. A	703. C	756. D
598. F	651. A	704. A	757. E
599. H	652. A	705. B	758. A
600. G	653. B	706. A	759. E
601. A	654. M	707. E	760. C
602. B	655. I	708. D	761. B
603. J	656. O	709. B	762. B
604. D	657. G	710. A	763. E
605. C	658. C	711. B	764. C
606. L	659. N	712. B	765. E
607. E	660. J	713. E	766. B
608. M	661. H	714. C	767. C
609. I	662. F	715. E	768. C
610. N	663. E	716. A	769. B
611. K	664. K	717. C	770. A
612. B	665. D	718. J	771. D
613. E	666. E	719. F	772. B
614. J	667. F	720. E	773. C
615. A	668. G	721. G	774. A
616. C	669. A	722. D	775. C
617. F	670. J	723. A	776. A
618. G	671. C	724. B	777. D
619. D	672. I	725. C	778. A
620. I	673. B	726. H	779. B
621. H	674. D	727. I	780. B
622. I	675. D	728. B	781. A
623. F	676. H	729. D	782. C
624. E	677. G	730. A	783. D
625. G	678. B	731. D	784. B
626. B	679. H	732. E	785. A
627. C	680. F	733. E	786. C
628. A	681. I	734. D	787. E
629. D	682. D	735. E	788. F
630. H	683. E	736. C	789. D
631. B	684. J	737. D	790. E
632. A	685. A	738. B	791. C
633. D	686. C	739. A	792. B
634. A	687. B	740. B	793. A
635. F	688. B	741. I	794. C
636. B	689. A	742. F	795. F
637. I	690. D	743. J	796. B
638. C	691. E	744. E	797. A
639. E	692. A	745. A	798. E
640. K	693. E	746. C	799. D
641. G	694. C	747. G	800. G

SECTION II

801. D	854. A
802. B	855. C
803. A	856. C
804. A	857. A
805. A	858. B
806. B	859. E
807. B	860. A
808. B	861. D
809. C	862. E
810. A	863. D
811. B	864. D
812. B	865. B
813. D	866. B
814. C	867. C
815. B	868. D
816. E	869. A
817. D	870. D
818. A	871. E
819. C	872. B
820. A	873. C
821. E	874. E
822. E	875. B
823. D	876. C
824. A	877. B
825. E	878. D
826. B	879. D
827. C	880. A
828. A	881. B
829. A	882. C
830. B	883. E
831. D	884. A
832. C	885. A
833. B	886. E
834. A	887. D
835. E	888. A
836. C	889. C
837. C	890. E
838. B	891. E
839. B	892. B
840. A	893. C
841. A	894. A
842. C	895. D
843. A	896. C
844. C	897. D
845. E	898. E
846. B	899. A
847. A	900. E
848. B	901. B
849. C	902. D
850. D	903. C
851. B	904. D
852. C	905. A
853. D	906. D

SECTION II

907. C	960. C	1013. B	1066. E	1119. E
908. A	961. B	1014. E	1067. D	1120. G
909. B	962. D	1015. A	1068. C	1121. B
910. D	963. A	1016. D	1069. A	1122. B
911. A	964. B	1017. C	1070. A	1123. A
912. D	965. E	1018. B	1071. C	1124. B
913. A	966. D	1019. A	1072. B	1125. E
914. B	967. A	1020. D	1073. D	1126. D
915. C	968. C	1021. D	1074. A	1127. C
916. B	969. A	1022. A	1075. C	1128. C
917. D	970. B	1023. E	1076. B	1129. E
918. D	971. D	1024. C	1077. C	1130. J
919. B	972. E	1025. A	1078. E	1131. A
920. A	973. C	1026. B	1079. F	1132. F
921. A	974. A	1027. D	1080. B	1133. G
922. C	975. B	1028. A	1081. A	1134. H
923. A	976. C	1029. E	1082. D	1135. B
924. A	977. D	1030. D	1083. I	1136. D
925. B	978. E	1031. C	1084. H	1137. I
926. D	979. A	1032. D	1085. G	1138. A
927. D	980. C	1033. A	1086. B	1139. B
928. D	981. B	1034. D	1087. C	1140. B
929. D	982. D	1035. D	1088. D	1141. A
930. E	983. E	1036. C	1089. A	1142. B
931. C	984. A	1037. A	1090. F	1143. A
932. D	985. C	1038. D	1091. E	1144. A
933. E	986. A	1039. E	1092. B	1145. C
934. C	987. D	1040. B	1093. A	1146. A
935. A	988. E	1041. C	1094. E	1147. A
936. C	989. B	1042. A	1095. D	1148. B
937. D	990. D	1043. E	1096. C	1149. E
938. C	991. A	1044. D	1097. C	1150. A
939. A	992. D	1045. D	1098. D	1151. F
940. D	993. C	1046. A	1099. B	1152. D
941. A	994. C	1047. E	1100. F	1153. C
942. C	995. D	1048. B	1101. E	1154. E
943. C	996. E	1049. C	1102. A	1155. G
944. D	997. A	1050. B	1103. G	1156. B
945. E	998. B	1051. C	1104. H	1157. D
946. C	999. B	1052. A	1105. C	1158. H
947. B	1000. A	1053. B	1106. D	1159. A
948. B	1001. C	1054. E	1107. A	1160. J
949. D	1002. E	1055. D	1108. B	1161. C
950. C	1003. D	1056. E	1109. F	1162. F
951. A	1004. E	1057. E	1110. E	1163. I
952. E	1005. D	1058. A	1111. G	1164. C
953. B	1006. E	1059. B	1112. D	1165. D
954. E	1007. B	1060. D	1113. F	1166. A
955. D	1008. A	1061. A	1114. A	1167. E
956. B	1009. C	1062. D	1115. A	1168. F
957. C	1010. E	1063. C	1116. A	1169. C
958. A	1011. D	1064. B	1117. B	1170. E
959. E	1012. C	1065. A	1118. C	1171. A

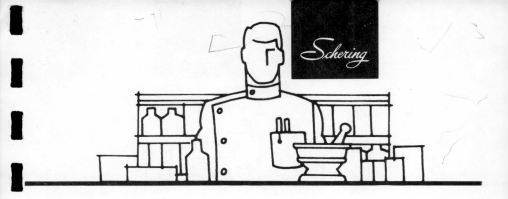

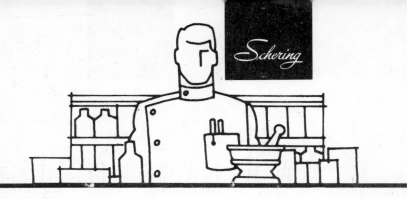

Quality Schering OTC products you can recommend with confidence

CORICIDIN ® Tablets–Maximum strength in a non-prescription product for temporary relief of cold or flu symptoms (runny nose, body aches, fever).

CORICIDIN 'D' ® Tablets–Same effective ingredients as regular CORICIDIN plus a decongestant to temporarily relieve nasal congestion due to colds, promote sinus drainage and restore freer nasal breathing.

CORICIDIN DEMILETS ® Tablets–Chewable, decongestant tablets for relief of children's stuffy and runny noses and other cold symptoms.

TINACTIN ® Solution and Cream–Kills athlete's foot and jock itch fungi on contact.

TINACTIN ® Powder and Powder Aerosol–Helps prevent athlete's foot re-infection.

AFRIN ® Nasal Spray/Nose Drops–The longest lasting topical nasal decongestant. Twice a day use provides up to 24 hour relief of nasal congestion due to colds, sinus congestion and hay fever.

CHLOR-TRIMETON ® Allergy Tablets 4mg./Syrup–A recognized standard for effective allergy treatment, where congestion is not a problem.

CHLOR-TRIMETON Decongestant Tablets–when sinus/nasal congestion complicates upper respiratory allergy.

'A and D' Hand Cream–Superior treatment for dry, chapped hands.
Reg TM

'A and D' Ointment–For quick, soothing relief of diaper rash, dry
Reg TM
chafed skin and minor burns in children and adults.

DEMAZIN ® Syrup–For temporary relief of nasal congestion due to hay fever and sinusitis.

DEMAZIN REPETABS ® Tablets–Long acting relief of nasal congestion due to hay fever and sinusitis.

Professionally Preferred–Professionally Recommended

SECTION II

1172. B	1222. A	1275. B	1328. B	1381. B
1173. D	1223. C	1276. D	1329. D	1382. C
1174. B	1224. D	1277. E	1330. A	1383. D
1175. C	1225. E	1278. A	1331. E	1384. A
1176. A	1226. B	1279. B	1332. A	1385. C
1177. E	1227. A	1280. C	1333. A	1386. E
1178. D	1228. B	1281. C	1334. C	1387. C
1179. A	1229. C	1282. C	1335. C	1388. B
1180. C	1230. D	1283. B	1336. D	1389. D
1181. B	1231. A	1284. D	1337. C	1390. E
1182. D	1232. E	1285. A	1338. A	1391. E
1183. E	1233. B	1286. C	1339. A	1392. A
1184. E	1234. D	1287. D	1340. A	1393. C
1185. D	1235. C	1288. C	1341. B	1394. D
1186. C	1236. A	1289. B	1342. B	1395. D
1187. D	1237. D	1290. A	1343. A	1396. C
1188. B	1238. C	1291. B	1344. B	1397. D
1189. E	1239. E	1292. A	1345. C	1398. C
1190. D	1240. D	1293. D	1346. D	1399. B
1191. A	1241. C	1294. C	1347. A	1400. A
1192. C	1242. A	1295. C	1348. B	1401. B
1193. A	1243. C	1296. D	1349. D	1402. A
1194. A	1244. B	1297. E	1350. C	1403. A
1195. D	1245. B	1298. E	1351. B	1404. B
1196. E	1246. B	1299. E	1352. A	1405. D
1197. C	1247. C	1300. E	1353. D	1406. C
1198. A	1248. A	1301. D	1354. D	1407. B
1199. E	1249. B	1302. A	1355. B	1408. B
1200. B	1250. D	1303. D	1356. B	1409. C
1201. D	1251. D	1304. B	1357. E	1410. A
1202. D	1252. C	1305. C	1358. D	1411. D
1203. E	1253. B	1306. D	1359. B	1412. E
1204. B	1254. A	1307. B	1360. A	1413. B
1205. B	1255. E	1308. C	1361. B	1414. A
1206. E	1256. A	1309. B	1362. B	1415. B
1207. E	1257. D	1310. B	1363. B	1416. C
1208. E	1258. D	1311. D	1364. E	1417. B
1209. C	1259. E	1312. D	1365. A	1418. A
1210. A	1260. B	1313. C	1366. C	1419. C
	1261. A	1314. D	1367. D	1420. B
	1262. A	1315. E	1368. D	1421. D
SECTION III	1263. E	1316. B	1369. A	1422. C
	1264. A	1317. D	1370. B	1423. D
1211. A	1265. E	1318. E	1371. E	1424. C
1212. C	1266. A	1319. D	1372. C	1425. B
1213. D	1267. A	1320. C	1373. C	1426. A
1214. B	1268. C	1321. D	1374. D	1427. D
1215. E	1269. A	1322. A	1375. E	1428. B
1216. D	1270. A	1323. C	1376. C	1429. B
1217. C	1271. D	1324. D	1377. A	1430. C
1218. A	1272. A	1325. E	1378. E	1431. A
1219. E	1273. E	1326. C	1379. A	1432. D
1220. D	1274. E	1327. D	1380. A	1433. D
1221. C				

SECTION III

1434. D	1484. A	1537. E	1590. B	1643. B
1435. C	1485. E	1538. A	1591. A	1644. A
1436. D	1466. C	1539. D	1592. C	1645. A
1437. B	1487. C	1540. E	1593. B	
1438. B	1488. A	1541. A	1594. E	**SECTION V**
1439. E	1489. C	1542. B	1595. D	
1440. B	1490. D	1543. A	1596. A	1646. C
1441. B	1491. A	1544. A	1597. C	1647. B
1442. D	1492. B	1545. A	1598. B	1648. B
1443. D	1493. A	1546. D	1599. D	1649. B
1444. B	1494. B	1547. B	1600. A	1650. A
1445. E	1495. B	1548. A	1601. E	1651. A
1446. E	1496. A	1549. C	1602. C	1652. D
1447. B	1497. D	1550. D	1603. C	1653. E
1448. C	1498. D	1551. H	1604. A	1654. D
1449. D	1499. A	1552. A	1605. B	1655. C
1450. D	1500. E	1553. F	1606. D	1656. C
1451. B	1501. C	1554. J	1607. E	1657. B
1452. A	1502. B	1555. B	1608. E	1658. D
1453. C	1503. D	1556. E	1609. D	1659. B
1454. B	1504. E	1557. C	1610. D	1660. C
1455. B	1505. C	1558. G	1611. C	1661. C
1456. B	1506. A	1559. I	1612. B	1662. D
1457. E	1507. B	1560. K	1613. A	1663. D
1458. B	1508. D	1561. L	1614. E	1664. C
1459. E	1509. E	1562. B	1615. F	1665. D
1460. C	1510. E	1563. B	1616. G	1666. B
1461. A	1511. D	1564. A	1617. E	1667. D
1462. C	1512. A	1565. C	1618. H	1668. D
1463. C	1513. B	1566. B	1619. B	1669. A
1464. C	1514. C	1567. B	1620. I	1670. C
1465. A	1515. B	1568. C	1621. A	1671. D
1466. B	1516. D	1569. A	1622. F	1672. E
1467. B	1517. C	1570. D	1623. C	1673. A
1468. B	1518. C	1571. B	1624. G	1674. D
1469. B	1519. D	1572. B	1625. J	1675. A
1470. D	1520. A	1573. E	1626. D	1676. E
	1521. B	1574. A	1627. A	1677. B
SECTION IV	1522. B	1575. C	1628. B	1678. B
	1523. C	1576. D	1629. A	1679. B
1471. B	1524. A	1577. F	1630. D	1680. C
1472. C	1525. C	1578. E	1631. C	1681. A
1473. C	1526. E	1579. D	1632. C	1682. D
1474. D	1527. E	1580. B	1633. C	1683. C
1475. B	1528. B	1581. C	1634. A	1684. D
1476. C	1529. B	1582. A	1635. C	1685. D
1477. C	1530. D	1583. C	1636. B	1686. D
1478. D	1531. C	1584. B	1637. B	1687. D
1479. C	1532. E	1585. C	1638. D	1688. E
1480. A	1533. A	1586. D	1639. B	1689. E
1481. C	1534. B	1587. E	1640. C	1690. B
1482. D	1535. C	1588. A	1641. C	1691. D
1483. B	1536. B	1589. C	1642. C	1692. C

SECTION V

1693. C	1746. E	1799. C	1849. A	1902. A
1694. A	1747. B	1800. C	1850. B	1903. B
1695. E	1748. D	1801. E	1851. B	1904. A
1696. D	1749. B	1802. E	1852. D	1905. D
1697. C	1750. A	1803. E	1853. D	1906. B
1698. B	1751. C	1804. A	1854. B	1907. C
1699. C	1752. C	1805. D	1855. A	1908. A
1700. C	1753. C	1806. D	1856. C	1909. F
1701. B	1754. E	1807. D	1857. E	1910. H
1702. A	1755. A	1808. A	1858. B	1911. D
1703. C	1756. A	1809. C	1859. D	1912. A
1704. C	1757. E	1810. E	1860. E	1913. B
1705. A	1758. A	1811. D	1861. C	1914. C
1706. C	1759. C	1812. D	1862. A	1915. G
1707. A	1760. D	1813. D	1863. A	1916. E
1708. C	1761. G	1814. B	1864. D	1917. D
1709. A	1762. F	1815. A	1865. A	1918. C
1710. E	1763. E	1816. D	1866. B	1919. B
1711. B	1764. B	1817. D	1867. A	1920. D
1712. D	1765. C	1818. C	1868. C	1921. D
1713. D	1766. C	1819. D	1869. E	1922. C
1714. C	1767. B	1820. A	1870. D	1923. D
1715. A	1768. C		1871. A	1924. C
1716. E	1769. E	**SECTION VI**	1872. A	1925. C
1717. B	1770. E		1873. C	1926. D
1718. B	1771. D	1821. A	1874. C	1927. E
1719. D	1772. C	1822. C	1875. D	1928. C
1720. A	1773. B	1823. C	1876. F	1929. D
1721. C	1774. B	1824. A	1877. G	1930. A
1722. E	1775. D	1825. E	1878. A	1931. D
1723. C	1776. A	1826. D	1879. B	1932. D
1724. D	1777. D	1827. C	1880. E	1933. B
1725. B	1778. C	1828. C	1881. B	1934. D
1726. C	1779. E	1829. A	1882. D	1935. B
1727. E	1780. A	1830. A	1883. E	1936. B
1728. E	1781. C	1831. C	1884. A	1937. D
1729. D	1782. C	1832. E	1885. C	1938. C
1730. E	1783. D	1833. A	1886. C	1939. A
1731. D	1784. B	1834. C	1887. B	1940. C
1732. B	1785. D	1835. A	1888. B	1941. C
1733. A	1786. E	1836. D	1889. D	1942. C
1734. C	1787. B	1837. A	1890. A	1943. B
1735. D	1788. A	1838. D	1891. B	1944. C
1736. D	1789. D	1839. B	1892. B	1945. C
1737. E	1790. D	1840. E	1893. C	1946. C
1738. D	1791. C	1841. D	1894. C	1947. B
1739. C	1792. C	1842. E	1895. B	1948. C
1740. A	1793. D	1843. A	1896. D	1949. B
1741. B	1794. D	1844. D	1897. A	1950. B
1742. E	1795. C	1845. A	1898. E	1951. C
1743. D	1796. B	1846. C	1899. C	1952. B
1744. D	1797. B	1847. D	1900. F	1953. C
1745. A	1798. A	1848. A	1901. B	1954. D

SECTION VI

1955. D	2008. A
1956. A	2009. C
1957. B	2010. B
1958. B	2011. A
1959. B	2012. D
1960. B	2013. E
1961. A	2014. C
1962. A	2015. C
1963. A	2016. A
1964. B	2017. E
1965. C	2018. C
1966. C	2019. C
1967. C	2020. C
1968. D	
1969. C	
1970. D	
1971. D	
1972. C	
1973. B	
1974. C	
1975. C	
1976. D	
1977. G	
1978. I	
1979. B	
1980. J	
1981. B	
1982. B	
1983. B	
1984. F	
1985. H	
1986. A	
1987. D	
1988. D	
1989. C	
1990. A	
1991. B	
1992. C	
1993. C	
1994. B	
1995. A	
1996. C	
1997. A	
1998. B	
1999. E	
2000. A	
2001. B	
2002. B	
2003. D	
2004. B	
2005. D	
2006. A	
2007. C	